CONTEMPORARY ISSUES IN THE U.S. HEALTHCARE DEBATE

ELISHA CALDWELL, MPH

authorHOUSE®

AuthorHouse™
1663 Liberty Drive
Bloomington, IN 47403
www.authorhouse.com
Phone: 1 (800) 839-8640

© 2019 Elisha Caldwell, MPH. All rights reserved.

No part of this book may be reproduced, stored in a retrieval system, or transmitted by any means without the written permission of the author.

Published by AuthorHouse 06/27/2019

ISBN: 978-1-7283-0944-6 (sc)
ISBN: 978-1-7283-0943-9 (e)

Print information available on the last page.

This book is printed on acid-free paper.

Because of the dynamic nature of the Internet, any web addresses or links contained in this book may have changed since publication and may no longer be valid. The views expressed in this work are solely those of the author and do not necessarily reflect the views of the publisher, and the publisher hereby disclaims any responsibility for them.

I am delighted to dedicate this book to my wife Monica Willie Caldwell and my three children Joyce M. Caldwell, Elisha A. Caldwell, Jr., and Darlington G. Caldwell for their endless support. It has been a great pleasure to have my family around me throughout my writing process.

CONTENTS

Abstract ix

Glossary xi

Introduction xiii

Historical Background of the U.S. Healthcare System 1

Drivers of U.S. High Healthcare Costs 19

References 93

ABSTRACT

Access to the United States (U.S.) healthcare system has been one of the contested debates in U.S. mainstream politics. The provision of access to medical services not only improves the mental and physical well-being of a population but also increases its lifespan, reduces years of potential lives lost, empowers the community, and subsequently leads to economic growth. Central to this core principle lies the World Health Organization's definition of health: a holistic dimension of physical, mental, and social well-being that constitutes the absence of disease or infirmity. At the core of the political upheaval in the United States—the election of President Donald J. Trump in 2016—ushered in an unprecedented move to adopt the American Healthcare Act of 2017. The impetus for this act was to repeal and replace the Patient Protection Affordable Care Act (ACA), penned into law in 2010 by Trump's predecessor, President Barack Obama. Although the majority-led Republican members of the House passed the Trump Care Act, it was authoritatively repealed by an unusual move by three Republicans who aligned with the Democrats. The failure of the American Healthcare Act to pass through the Senate was a significant milestone in the U.S. healthcare debate; proponents of the ACA could once again choose their own healthcare plan through the ACA.

GLOSSARY

AAMC Association of American Medical Colleges
ACA Affordable Care Act
AHA American Hospital Association
AHCA American Healthcare Act
AMA American Medical Association
CBO Congressional Budget Office
CDC Centers for Disease Control and Prevention
CHIP Children's Health Insurance Plan
CMS Centers for Medicare & Medicaid Services
EHR electronic health record
EHS entrepreneurial market-based insurance
FDA Food and Drug Administration
GDP gross domestic product
GOP Grand Old Party
NHE national healthcare expenditure
NHS National Health Service
OECD Organization for Economic Co-operation and Development
PDP prescription drug plan
PHE personal health expenditure

PRB Population Reference Bureau
RN registered nurse
SHI social health insurance
SS Social Security
UK United Kingdom
WHO World Health Organization

INTRODUCTION

The healthcare system in the United States seems fragile for its many actors: shareholders, stakeholders, and government and state entities. Despite these fragilities, the healthcare system has evolved since the Great Depression in the 1930s, beginning with the adoption of Social Security (SS) and continuing in the creation of Medicare and Medicaid in 1965 (American College of Healthcare Executives, n.d.). The United States is known for its expertise in biomedicine. It houses some of the world's most renowned experts in the field of medicine, public health, biomedical research, and the pharmaceutical industry. The United States is, by far, the biggest spender on healthcare per capita and gross domestic product (GDP; Organization for Economic Co-operation and Development [OECD], 2018). The U.S. modern healthcare infrastructure is unmatched. In the United States, most healthcare providers want to be based in its industrial structure with a high income. Despite these unequivocal characteristics, the United States remains the only advanced country in the world that has faced opposition from public opinion, lobbyists, and right-wing political activists in attempts to adopt universal access to healthcare.

The process of the U.S. healthcare delivery system has been extremely costly and fragmented by many federal and state actors and non-state actors including private insurance companies and pharmaceutical companies, at the expense of the very people who receive care: the patients. The sophisticated model manipulated and influenced by private companies has exerted pressure on a system that needs to be reinvigorated. The invasion of private companies into the U.S. healthcare system, as a result of competition at the beginning of the 1930s, has unveiled increasingly unavoidable and unaffordable access to care. The imbalance in this system has manifested in a corridor of mild poverty for so many Americans who are caught up in the so-called American Dream with unpaid medical bills in collections. As the demand for medical services increases in the United States, so does the cost and the price of a medical education.

U.S. national healthcare expenditures (NHEs) exceed $3.6 trillion a year, about 18% of its GDP (Centers for Medicare and Medicaid Services [CMS], 2018; World Bank, 2018; CIA World Factbook, 2018; WHO, n.d.). The NHE budget surpasses the GDP of most G7 countries including Canada ($1.8 trillion), the United Kingdom ($2.94 trillion), and France ($2.93 trillion). The G7 countries are the world's super-rich that adopts policies on pressing issues like security, economies, and energy, to smooth global cooperation. Despite this massive spending, access to healthcare at the microlevel has been uneven for decades in the United States. The industrialization that took place in the United States, coupled with public health interventions decades ago in the 20th century, promoted population health. Then, the United States shifted through a cycle of epidemiological transitions, demonstrating that infectious diseases that once were the cause of ill-health and death were replaced by chronic diseases like cancer, diabetes, obesity, and stroke, among others (Center for Disease Control and Prevention [CDC], 2017). At the core of the healthcare debate, healthcare reform could be a zero-sum game if those in the top positions are not well informed about healthcare policy. At the microlevel (the hospital setting), reform in the healthcare industry can have negative and positive impacts on patient-health outcomes. The debate on healthcare reform in the United States should start with reform in the pharmaceutical industry, a rational political gesture from policymakers, very powerful lobbyists that have longstanding opposition to reform, the American Medical Association (AMA) and the American Hospital Association (AHA).

HISTORICAL BACKGROUND OF THE U.S. HEALTHCARE SYSTEM

The U.S. healthcare system has evolved over time, beginning with the introduction of SS, signed into law by President Franklin D. Roosevelt and the 74th Congress in 1935 (American College of Healthcare Executives, n.d.). The birth of SS fell short in addressing the health needs of the U.S. population at the time. As the U.S. economy began to take shape, drowning out the Great Depression, the issue of health insurance constituted a heated debate in the 1930s. Physicians, providers, and hospitals expressed concern about the inability of patients to pay for services. This marked the beginning of today's Medicare and Medicaid and the advent of private and commercial insurance in the market. In 1965, after a gruesome debate in both houses, a bill that became known as Medicare and Medicaid was pen into law by President Lyndon B, Johnson (American College of Healthcare Executives, n.d.; CMS, 2018). Since its inception more than five decades ago, Medicare evolved to provide health insurance for disabled individuals diagnosed with end-stage renal disease, and seniors 65 years and older. Despite the introduction of Medicare, many Americans were left without any type of health insurance. As the U.S. population increased over time, much of the population was not at an age to qualify for Medicare. Increasingly, a large portion of the population had income above the threshold to qualify for Medicaid and the Children's Health Insurance Plan (CHIP) but had too little income to afford private insurance. This financial drain left millions of the U.S. population in limbo, wandering in the healthcare system uninsured. The government had little to offer them until 2010 when President Obama's sweeping legislation, the Patient Protection and Affordable Care Act, was signed into law. This was a moment that brought the United States ever closer to universal health access to care. Although the ACA engenders many challenges, it has afforded the U.S. population the choice to choose their own healthcare plan.

Cost of Medical School

The United States is known for its expertise in biomedicine. It houses one of the world's renowned experts in the field of biomedicine and scientific research. The United States has an open-door policy. Medical schools in the United States admit students from around the world. This innovative approach has unleashed a remarkably nurturing power in the scientific community: a community of diversity, and leadership. Despite these recognizable characteristics of the U.S. medical scientific community, it has had a tradition of resistance to government-sponsored health insurance programs since the Great Depression, based on income (American College of Healthcare Executives, n.d.).

As the demand for medical services increases in the United States, so does the cost and the price to train medical professionals. The cost of medical school has incrementally expanded since the 1980s. As described by the Association of American Medical Colleges (AAMC), the cost of medical tuition was approximately $30,000 for private school and $20,000 for a public school in the first year in figure 1. These figures are estimates and could differ on a case-by-case basis that is entirely at the schools' discretion. However, students were not required to purchase insurance.

Statistics from the AAMC shows 860,917 active physicians in all specialties in 2015; of those, 577, 313 were active U.S. physicians (AAMC, 2015). A recent report from the Kaiser Family Foundation (2018) demonstrated an increase of practicing physician in all specialties, with a national average of 968,743, of whom 467, 447 work in primary care. According to the U.S. Bureau of Labor Statistics, the occupational outlook in the medical field is promising. The education platform for a physician, set forth as described by the Bureau of Labor Statistics (2018), requires a bachelor degree, four years of study at a medical school, and 3 to 7 years of residency or internship aligned with the specialty requirement to be qualified. Although the need for healthcare professionals has increased over time in the United States, the cost of obtaining a medical education has increasingly become costly and unaffordable. The cost of medical school has evolved over the past few decades, as illustrated in Figure 1 for tuition and fees for first-year medical students from 1996 to 1997 compared to Figure 2, assessing the period from 2017 to 2018.

Figure 1: Tuition for first-year medical students 1996–1997

Source: Association of American Medical College

Academic Year	Cost Type	Ownership Type	Residence Status	Minimum Cost	Median Cost	Maximum Cost	Average Cost	Average Cost Percent Change from Prior Year
1996-1997	Tuition and Fees	Public	Resident	$0	$9,097	$20,129	$9,779	4.9%
1996-1997	Tuition and Fees	Private	Resident	$8,152	$24,963	$31,925	$24,002	5.9%
1996-1997	Tuition and Fees	Public	Nonresident	$0	$20,806	$51,669	$21,582	6.1%
1996-1997	Tuition and Fees	Private	Nonresident	$16,400	$25,212	$31,925	$25,395	5.3%

Figure 2: Tuition for first-year medical students 2017–2018

Source: Association of American Medical College

Academic Year	Cost Type	Ownership Type	Residence Status	Minimum Cost	Median Cost	Maximum Cost	Average Cost	Average Cost Percent Change from Prior Year
2017-2018	Tuition, Fees, and Health Insurance	Public	Resident	$0	$36,809	$53,327	$35,704	3.2%
2017-2018	Tuition, Fees, and Health Insurance	Private	Resident	$24,363	$59,466	$86,661	$57,194	2.9%
2017-2018	Tuition, Fees, and Health Insurance	Public	Nonresident	$0	$62,434	$98,538	$60,141	2.4%
2017-2018	Tuition, Fees, and Health Insurance	Private	Nonresident	$37,165	$60,245	$67,480	$58,709	3.2%

Figure 1 shows that during the late 1990s, private medical schools were charging freshman medical students a maximum tuition and fees of about $20,129 for in-state students and $51,669 for out-of-state students. In contrast to public colleges, the maximum cost for tuition and fees for a residential and nonresidential student in their first year in private schools was $31,925. The average cost of tuition and fees for a public medical school for in-state students was $9,779, with an estimated $21,582 for out-of-state students. During this era, medical students were not required to purchase insurance as part of their tuition and fees or separately. As schools opened to the global market, medical schools became increasingly expensive, competitive, and innovative. Medical schools in the United States admit students from the global community who are bright and able to make a significant contribution to the medical field.

As the field of biomedicine evolves, so does the cost. Medical schools began charging first-year students mandatory insurance in addition to the cost of tuition. The average cost of tuition, fees, and insurance for sophomore medical students considered residential (in-state) for public schools in 2017–2018 was $35,704; triple the tuition and fees charged in the 1990s. Private resident students paid an average cost of $57,194 for tuition, fees, and health insurance, shown in Figure 2, compared to the $24,002 shown in Figure 1. In contrast to resident students, nonresident students in public schools (see Figure 2) paid $60,141 on average for tuition, fees, and health insurance. Nonresident students in private schools had an average cost for tuition, fees, and health insurance of $58,709; double the cost of tuition and fees in 1990s. More alarming is the maximum cost medical schools could charge first-year medical students. As shown in Figure 1, the maximum cost for a resident student in a public college was $20,129 in the 1990s; half the maximum cost of tuition, fees, and health insurance ($53,327) charged in 2017 and 2018. In a similar vein, the maximum cost for tuition, fees, and insurance in 2017 and 2018 for nonresidents in public school was $98,538, quadrupling the charge in the 1990s.

As the U.S. healthcare system becomes technologically friendly and innovative and draws talented medical students from home and abroad, mandatory health insurance and the high cost of tuition and fees has become commonplace. The cost of medical school is becoming increasingly unattractive to many who wish to pursue a career in this field. As the data in Figures 1 and 2 propose, by the time a medical student reaches their fourth year and is ready to graduate, those who are on student loans will accumulate significant debt. Most of these students will require additional training for a specialization with the expectation of earning more to keep up with the demand of their student loans and the cost of living.

Despite the high cost of medical school in the United States, the occupational outlook in the biomedical field seems to be lucrative and promising. According to the U.S. Bureau of Labor Statistics (2018), the biomedical field is one of the fastest growing occupations in the United States. It is estimated that the career prospect for physicians and surgeons will increase by 13% from 2016 to 2026. In 2017, the median pay for a physician in the United States was $100 per hour for those taking salaries greater than or equal to $208,000 per year.

As the field of biomedicine progressively overtook most of the occupation, records show 713,800 jobs in this field in 2016, with an increase of 91,400 projected by 2026 (U.S. Bureau of Labor Statistics, 2018). The field of Western medicine, as biomedicine is often referenced, has involved in the 21st century to include multiple disciplines. Some captivating professions in biomedicine dubbed attractive occupations are anesthesiologist, surgeon, obstetrician and gynecologist, psychiatrist, family and general medicine, general internist, and pediatrician. The annual income of doctors in these professions, according to data from the U.S. Bureau of Labor Statistics (2017) are displayed in Figures 3 and 4. The career outlook in the anesthesiology specialty in the U.S. biomedical field reports higher pay in 2017 (see Figure 3). Anesthesiologists had the highest pay in 2017. They had an estimated income of $265,990, surpassing those in other disciplines in the field of biomedicine, as depicted in Figure 3. As reported by the U.S. Bureau of Labor Statistics (2018), Figure 4 depicts that those in biomedicine have a higher median income than those in most occupations in the U.S. economy.

Figure 3: Income by discipline in biomedicine

Source: US Bureau of Labor Statistics

Anesthesiologists	$265,990
Surgeons	251,890
Obstetricians and gynecologists	235,240
Psychiatrists	216,090
Physicians and surgeons, all other	211,390
Family and general practitioners	208,560
Internists, general	198,370
Pediatricians, general	187,540

Figure 4: Physicians and surgeons median annual income

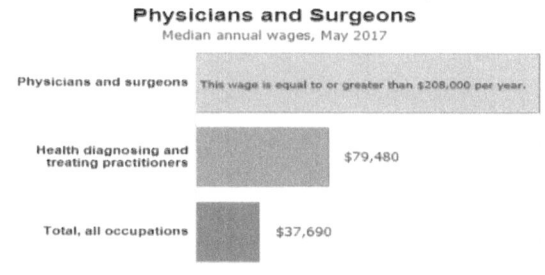

It is not surprising that, in the United States, as the demand for healthcare workers proliferates, income and training for professionals in the biomedical field increases as well. This relationship can create stress on the healthcare system. According to the Population Reference Bureau (PRB, 2017), the U.S. population has reached 329.3 million people, the third most populous country in the world, following China and India. According to PRB statistics, the U.S. total fertility rate has steadily declined since the earlier 2000s. In 2016, according to PRB, U.S. total fertility rate reached a record low of 1.82 children per woman, shown in Figure 5. It is crucially important to understand the population, growth, change, and dynamics to build a sustainable healthcare system. Although the U.S. population has become more diverse and is aging, population change from 2010 to 2017 was about 5.3%, a decrease from 9.6% from 2000 to 2010 (PRB, 2017). As society aged, the demand for medical facilities, direct care, and senior living centers become inevitable. As chronicled by the PRB (2017), the United States has 15.2% of its populations aged 65 and above. Nearly 22.8% of the U.S. population is younger than 18 years of age. The United States has gone through an epidemiological transition. Chronic disease has become predominant in society and could affect the aging population's ability to become effective and efficient in managing their state of health. Figure 6 establishes the percentage of U.S. seniors' (65+) structure and how it has gradually surged upwards since the 2000s.

Figure 5: US total fertility rate

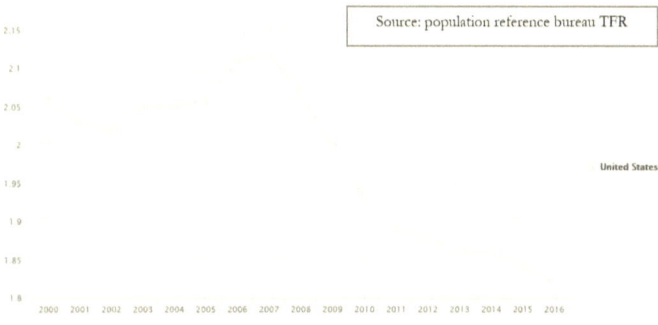

Figure 6: Percentage of the US population ages 65 and older

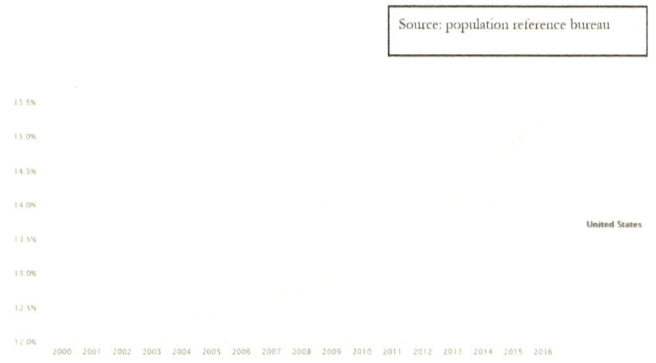

Nurses

Nurses are angels in the U.S. healthcare system. They comprise a significant part of the healthcare workforce. Students do not require 5 to 10 years of school to become a registered nurse (RN); rather, one can achieve a traditional Bachelor of Science in nursing degree in 4 years, an associate degree in nursing in 2 years, or take part in an approved program that issues diplomas in nursing (U.S. Bureau of Labor Statistics, 2018). All nurses are required by law to be certified through the National Council of States Boards of Nursing.

Nurses usually spend more time with patients and have greater direct-care responsibilities than physicians. The degree of education, license, practice, and salary between nurses and physicians differs significantly. Nurses must employ critical-thinking skills to deter the poor health of a patient. The absence of physical illness does not rule out the need for help to attain well-being and a good state of mind. Nurses should be alert at all times. Nurses should be good communicators, compassionate, detail oriented, emotionally stable, organized, and physically and mentally stable (U.S. Bureau of Labor Statistics, 2018.

The career outlook in the field of nursing is favorable in the United States, particularly for those who want to move beyond the RN degree, obtaining a master's degree or Ph.D. Nurses have myriad opportunities and the prospect of acquiring a job after graduation is high. The field of nursing is expected to grow by 15% (U.S. Bureau of Labor Statistics, 2018). In 2017, RNs had a median income of $70,000. Of course, median income can be determined by employment facility, geography, and experiences. Figure 7 shows RNs have the potential to grow further than any those in any other career field in the U.S. economy. Those with specializations in health diagnosis and treating practitioners could see a growth of 16% from 2016, whereas the field of RNs is expected to be 15% in that time period.

Figure 7: Career Projection in Nursing Field

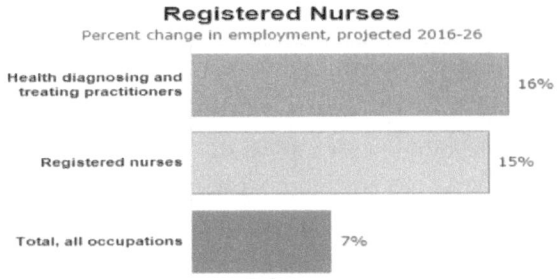

Pharmacists

At the core of the U.S. healthcare workforce are pharmacists. The pharmaceutical industry characterizes a significant part of the U.S. healthcare system. In most cases, in the United States one can obtain medicine in two common ways: an individual provider prescribing medication or at a pharmacy for medicine that does not require a provider prescription. In either way the medication must be manufactured by pharmaceutical companies, regulated by the Food and Drugs Administration (FDA). Although the FDA regulates drugs from clinical trials to marketing, some over-the-counter medications indicate on the label that the medication not been verified by the FDA. Regardless of this statement, the pharmaceutical company and pharmacist will sell their drugs.

Although the occupational outlook of pharmacists might not be fast growing in number of jobs compared to nurses and physicians, it is lucrative. The median pay for a pharmacist in 2017 was $124,170 (U.S. Bureau of Labor Statistics, 2018). Becoming a pharmacist should be an individual choice. However, with the U.S. population aging, the slow pace of growth in this area will require investment in training the next generation. Educational training for pharmacists entails 2 to 4 years of college coursework and roughly 4 years of doctorate work and an examination to be licensed as Pharm.D. Pharmacists are expected to possess a high quality of analysis, communication, technology, management, and organizational skills (U.S. Bureau of Labor Statistics, 2018).

What does this mean for the U.S. aging population?

One must not be misled by the wealth of medical professionals the United States produces each year and the extravagant spending on health to think that Americans are the healthiest population on earth. Unquestionably, the United States is preeminent in allocating monetary resources to healthcare. However, its population faces chronic medical conditions that lead to years of potential life difficulties and many lives lost. Figure 8 displays the characteristics of the U.S. population. The ages between 25 and 55 years is clustered in the middle of the graph, suggesting the United States has a fairly young population. When focused on the U.S. fertility rate, population change, and annual growth rate, the United States has a population of 329.3 million people; the third largest population in the world, following China and India (U.S. Census Bureau, 2017). The annual population growth rate from 2017 to 2018 was 0.80 with a declining total fertility rate of 1.9; the current life expectancy is 80.1 years (U.S. Census Bureau, 2017; CDC, 2017). As the U.S. population ages, chronic disease has taken a heavy toll on the population. Reports from the CDC (2017) suggest that heart disease, cancer, chronic lower respiratory disease, accidents, stroke, Alzheimer, diabetes, influenza and pneumonia, nephritis, nephrotic syndrome, nephrosis, and intentional self-harm (suicide) are the leading causes of deaths in the United States. An estimated 2,712,630 deaths occur each year (CDC, 2017) with an infant mortality rate of 5.90 deaths per 1,000 live births (U.S. Census Bureau, 2017; CDC, 2017).

Figure 8: US population Pyramid

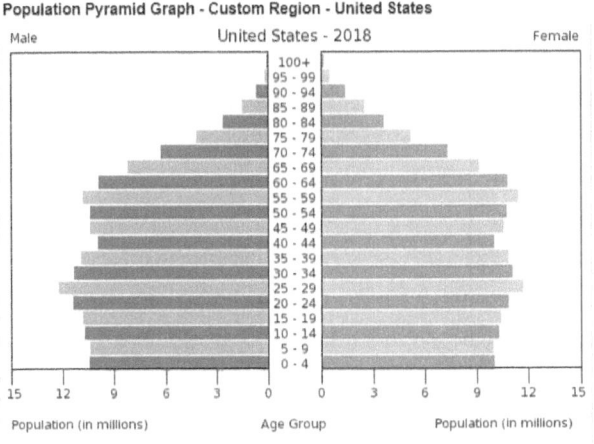

Healthcare professionals, particularly those in the medical field, enjoy the glamour of the U.S. workforce economy without any sign of plummeting. The medical profession has been a lucrative business and will outgrow other professions as the U.S. population fertility rate declines. The need for geriatric facilities will increase along with the demand for a geriatric healthcare workforce. Although not unique in a multicultural workforce, the United States may not be short of health professionals as it recruits competent individuals from across the globe.

Although this global integration has recently been under siege by the election of Donald J. Trump in 2016, it is arguably a short-term effect. Unlike the homogenous aging workforce in a country like Japan, the United States has benefited significantly from a diverse global scientific community and will likely continue in that vein. The unprecedented effects of Mr. Trump, who has displayed traits of a dictator and demonstrated lack of understanding of the global scientific community results in anxiety, fear, and ferocity among his right-wing idealist base that should not be ignored. The federalization of Trump's business mind in his political ideology under the pretext of loyalty, now embedded in the Grand Old Party (GOP), demonstrates a clear inconsistency with the U.S. constitution that was constructed on the principles of the right and will of the people. Despite these nonsensical impulses from Trump, the Republican establishment has undoubtedly supported Trump's poor policies on healthcare and trade, with the exception of the late Senator John McCain and other well-informed Republican lawmakers. The introduction of Trump's doctrine into Republican mainstream politics is a threat to the American long-standing ideology of democracy, the right to choose, and freedom of the press.

In spite of Trump's poor judgment, one must be mindful of any predictions about the 2020 presidential elections.

Central to the core of the political discontentment and divorce among the GOP elite club has been the attempted dismantlement of the Affordable Care Act (ACA) in 2017. The GOP has become a political football with many novice players. A controversial businessman who has never held public office or penned any healthcare policy in his lifetime ran his 2016 campaign platform on the pretext of repealing and replacing the ACA, if elected. This was an incredible reversal for a gifted man who knew how to deceive his base, manipulate public interest, disavow the late war hero Senator John McCain, and raise public anger, pronounced winner as the 45th President of the United States.

On numerous occasions, Mr. Trump did what he is best known for: manipulating well-respected GOP leaders like Paul Rayan and Mitch McConnell to repeal and replace the ACA. A disoriented act, known as the American Healthcare Act (AHCA) of 2017 was Mr. Trump's and the GOP's healthcare bill that passed the House of Representative, ignoring Congressional Budget Office (CBO) projections. Although the analysis from the CBO and the Joint Committee on Taxation indicated that if H.R. 1628 was to be in effect, the federal deficit would diminish by $119 billion from 2017 to 2026, an estimated 14 million Americans would go without insurance by 2018. When the AHCA reached the Senate floor for a final vote in 2017, a long-term critic of Mr. Trump, the late Senator John McCain from Arizona, along with two informed Republicans, Senator Susan Collins from Maine and Senator Lisa Murkowski from Alaska, aligned with the Democrats to repeal Trump's unpopular bill on healthcare. This was a milestone and a sense of hope that once again, constituents remain hopeful in those who represent them.

As a giant in healthcare, the U.S. NHE has reached a record high, $3.6 trillion, about 18% of U.S. GDP (International Monetary Fund, 2018; CMS, 2018; World Bank, 2018; CIA World Factbook, 2018; WHO, n.d.). The NHE surpasses the GDP of most G7 countries including Canada ($1.8 trillion), the United Kingdom ($2.94 trillion), and France ($2.93 trillion). The G7 countries are the world's super rich, adopting policies on pressing issues like security, economics, and energy that smooth global cooperation. This group of elites had eight members including Russia. Russia was thrown out in 2014, due to its annexation of Crimea in eastern Ukraine.

Russia ranked the 11th biggest economy in the global market (International Monetary Fund, 2018) and a world super power, sharing equitable amounts of nuclear arms race with the United States. Its ambitions in global geopolitics have increasingly become widely spread in places where U.S. policy has failed. Russia cannot be ignored in global politics. The core cause of Russia's membership of G7 being terminated was an interesting turning point in global politics. International law and order were actively manipulated, organized, and executed by U.S. unilateral policy in recent decades. The U.S. invasion of Iraq after 9/11 was a breach of international law. However, the U.S. G8 membership at the time was not suspended or terminated. In sharp contrast, of G8 members' troops, excluding their adversary Russia, fought shoulder to shoulder in Iraq and Afghanistan with U.S. troops. Russia has known for decades that the United

States does not abide by the rules in international politics, despite its track record in championing global democracy. The wealth of the United States has been its power, which is beyond the scope of this book. Figure 9 displays the GDP of G7 member states showing the advantage of the United States, leading other industrialized countries.

Figure 9: Gross domestic product, current prices (U.S. dollars)

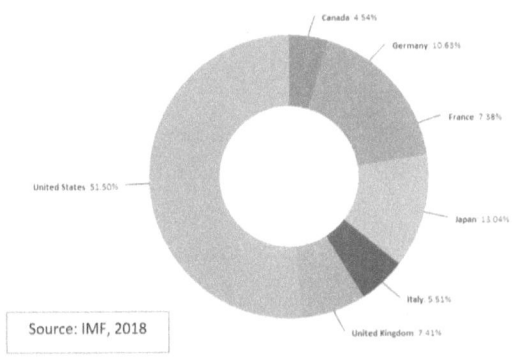

The United States is an economic giant and highly industrialized. Its GDP per capita and GDP share outweigh the rest of G7 member states. The United States has taken the bold step of outspending other wealthy countries on healthcare. However, one can only wish this excessive spending would make the U.S. populations healthier than those in other industrialized countries that use their resources smartly. The U.S. medical system is an island of fantasy that seems to be carefully crafted by smart individuals. These experts have been influenced by political ideology that affects millions of poor Americans or so-called working-class families. These families live in mild poverty in that they have enough to survive but not enough to attain the classic lifestyle in wealthy America. The government has cleverly determined how the health system should operate by using subdivision insurance schemes that target populations according to their needs since the 1930s. These subdivisions have evolved over time following the adoption of Medicare and Medicaid in the 1960s to include CHIP, and private insurance companies that complicate the system. Figure 10 shows the GDP per capita in G7 member states, once again showing the United States taking the lead.

Figure 10: Gross domestic product per capita, current prices (U.S. dollars)

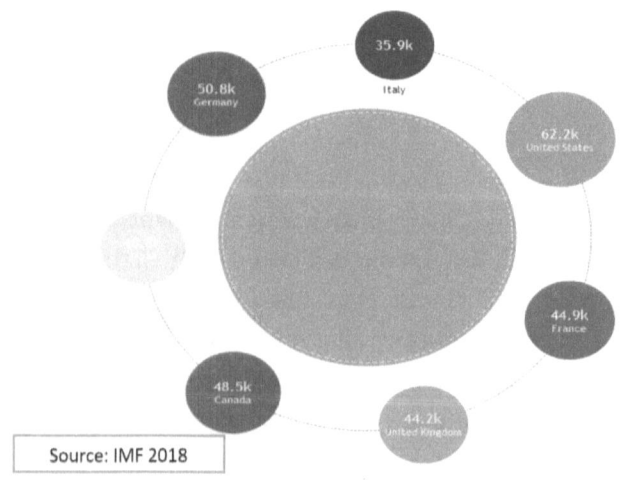

DRIVERS OF U.S. HIGH HEALTHCARE COSTS

Medicare: Since it was penned into law in the 1960s, Medicare has been costly. Seniors who are nearing retirement age have no idea if a reduced form of Medicare exists. The majority of senior citizens wait for the traditional retirement age of 65. Why wait this long when you have saved all your life for Medicare. In a similar vein, it is difficult for most retirees to navigate the three parts of Medicare. Medicare is part of the government affordable-insurance scheme that covers the cost of medical services for qualified individuals. It has three parts: Parts A, B, and D.

The government is crafty. Instead of creating a single system, it has overwhelmed the system with so many subsidies. To be qualified for Medicare one must be 1) 65 years or older, or 2) have some type of disability that Medicare deems qualified if you are under the age of 65. The exclusion and inclusion criteria are at the discretion of those who run Medicare.

In November every four years, a new government is elected in the United States. The new government takes office in January of the following year. Due do checks and balances, the new government is required to submit its annual budget to the CBO for analysis and projection before it can be submitted to Congress and to the U.S. public. Included in this review is the budget on healthcare for congressional review. Members of the CBO are not Democrats or Republicans; they are an independent agency that has the responsibility for free and fair analysis. These are experts. Their decision is not influenced by political ideology. Figure 11 describes the CBO's (2018) analysis of major healthcare expenditures.

Figure 11: CBO projection on major healthcare plan in 2018

PROJECTIONS FOR MAJOR HEALTH CARE PROGRAMS FOR FY 2018
(As of April 1, 2018)

MEDICARE (Net of Offsetting Receipts)	583 Billion
MEDICAID	383 Billion
HEALTH INSURANCE SUBSIDIES AND RELATED SPENDING	$58 Billion
CHILDREN'S HEALTH INSURANCE PROGRAM	$16 Billion

Source: Congressional Budget Office

How Much Money is Spent on Medicare

The NHE has an estimated budget of $3.6 trillion, roughly $10,348 per person (CMS, 2018). In other words, a single family's annual income may be close to the federal poverty line but will be diverted to healthcare. The CMS suggests that in 2016 Medicare expenditures surged to 3.6%, about $672.1 billion, and accounted for 20% of the NHE budget. If the current pace of healthcare expenditures continue, CMS projects the NHE budget will dramatically increase at a rate of 5.5% annually until 2026, burgeoning from $3.6 trillion to $5.5 trillion. The need for Medicare will nearly double to 7.4% and GDP expenditures on healthcare will also rise 19.7% (CMS, 2018).

How Many Americans Use Medicare

According to the Kaiser Family Foundation (2018), in 2015 a total of 55,504,004 Americans were receiving healthcare through Medicare. In the 50 states, five states had massive use of Medicare compared to other states: New York, California, Florida, Pennsylvania, and Texas, shown in Figures 12 and 13.

Figure 12: five states with large population of Medicare beneficiaries

Location	Total Medicare Beneficiaries
United States	55,504,005 [1]
California	5,644,384
Florida	4,024,223
New York	3,343,349
Pennsylvania	2,533,515
Texas	3,633,785

Figure 13: Medicare utilization by States

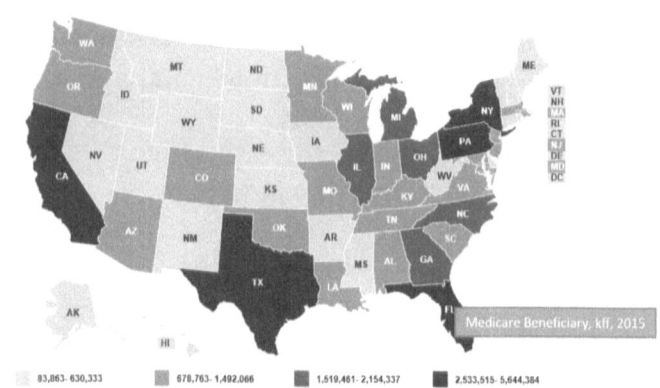

The uneven use of Medicare shown in Figure 13 is evidently found in the U.S. demographic structure. Before attempting to explore this further, it is vital to understand the demographics of these five states with the highest number of Medicare beneficiaries. The United States has an estimated 329.5 million people (U.S. Census Bureau, n.d; CIA World Factbook, 2018). According to the U.S. Census Bureau (n.d), an estimated 12.7% of the U.S. population lives in poverty. The five most populous states in the United States are California (39,188,300), Texas (27,677,200), Florida (20,545,300), New York (19,482,300) and Illinois (12,602,400; Kaiser Family Foundation, 2016). Pennsylvania narrowly lags behind Illinois in population and is one of the biggest consumers of Medicare. As the data suggest, the most populous states are more likely to have a high rate of Medicare users (excluding Illinois). The demographic characteristics of these states are also alike.

Although the U.S. population has become diverse over time, White people continue to dominate its population.

Nearly 76% of the populations are White (U.S. Census Bureau, n.d; CIA World Factbook, 2018). White Medicare beneficiaries across the United States differ substantially from non-White beneficiaries, raising a question about social-welfare programs and remains an area to explore. Although White people are main Medicare beneficiaries, that does not mean the system favors them. It could be because of White beneficiaries are the largest population. Figures 14, 15, and 16 display the percentage of Medicare consumers by race and ethnicity.

Figure 14: Percentage of Medicare Utilization by Whites

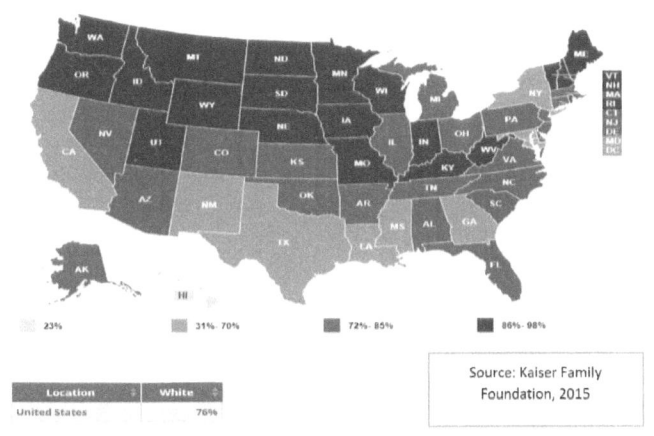

Source: Kaiser Family Foundation, 2015

Location	White
United States	76%

Figure 15: Percentage of Medicare Use by Blacks

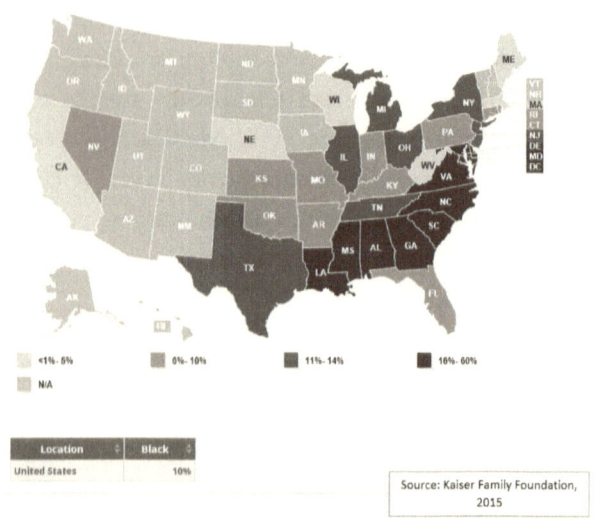

Source: Kaiser Family Foundation, 2015

Figure 16: Percentage of Medicare Use by Hispanics

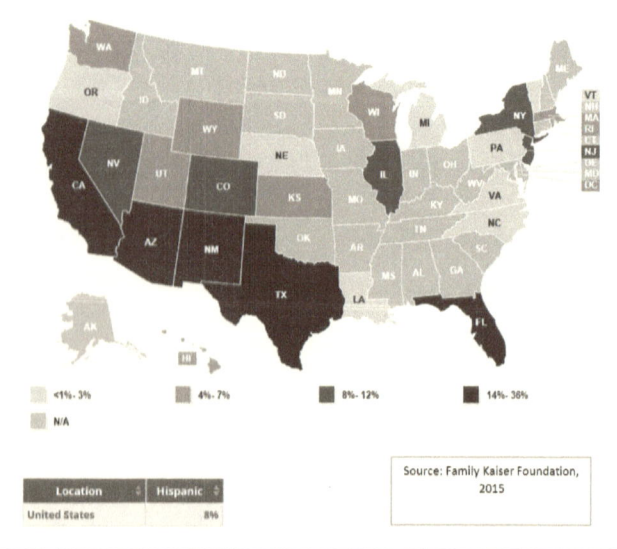

Source: Family Kaiser Foundation, 2015

Medicare use by race and ethnicity, shown on the three maps, is quite intriguing. Figure 14 shows that the majority of the 76% of the White people benefiting from Medicare are concentrated in the mid-central and northern part of the country. In contrast, Figure 15 shows a large number of the Black recipients are from the east coast and the deep South of the country. The bulk of the Hispanic community, according to the map in Figure 16 lies on the west coast. Any policy affecting Medicare should consider these maps.

Is it Worth the Cost—Why Should You be 65 or Have Preconditions to Qualify for Medicare

Prior to the inception of the ACA in 2010, the U.S. government has been ineffective in the insurance-market system. Although it has made some remarkable gains in public health, policymakers' refusals to make healthcare reform for all is undoubtedly caused by cowardness. The wealth of the United States is unmatched to the preconditions of its citizens and their access to affordable healthcare. The democratic system in the United States has fallen short in ensuring the health of the nation. In November every two years and every four years, voters go to the polls with policies in mind. Voting is an investment. To vote is to invest in one's desired candidate to represent their views. Unfortunately, Washington has turned into a cruise ship with a novice captain. The effect has been comparable to the Titanic, where everyone has turned to their political party for survivorship. The backlash from this kind of fault in a democratic system can be hugely catastrophic. These relentless political ideologies that have never been seen before in U.S. history will ruin the health of its citizen, if Washington continues to uphold its double standard. Healthcare should be a democratic right, like voting and should never be a precondition. Before you cast your vote to align with your interests, ask yourself why you vote. Does my voice matter in Washington? One thing you know is that every representative you send to Washing has access to good healthcare for themselves and their family. Do you and your family matter?

Access to care has been so politicized and so far has become aligned with political parties rather than with American ideals. Unless in the rare case one can be exempted from a tax deduction, every American contributes money from their income toward Medicare and Social Security. The deductions are made before a taxpayer gets their pay. Most taxpayers might not be aware of how much these deductions can be. It is worth looking at the paper or electronic pay stub to understand these deductions.

Most people living outside the United States might not realize that poverty exists in the United States. The United States is one of the unequal societies in the world. According to the OECD (2016), the United States had a Gini coefficient of 0.39 with a 0.178 poverty ratio in 2016. The U.S. poverty ratio is highest of all OCED member states. High levels of income differentials in any part of the world can undermine human rights and threaten the democratic system. The 2017 UN report on poverty in the United States suggested that nearly 40 million Americans are living in extreme poverty. The so-called working-class family in the United States is caught up in wealthy America's so-called American dream. They work hard but cannot get ahead. The U.S. tax system is skewed in favor of the wealthiest 1% and disproportionally affects the poor 50%. The government collects Medicare dollars and asks citizens to wait until they are 65 or have some disability to be eligible for benefits. Even at 65 years, Medicare eligibility subsidies are processed and not all forms of healthcare are covered. The issue of Medicare has become an ethical concern. Consider it this way: U.S. citizens begin to pay for Medicare as soon as they hold their first job. It is an expansive investment that is worth the care. However, by the standard average lifespan of most Americans, they will benefit from Medicare for only 10 years. The life expectancy for an average American is 78.6 years from birth, provided they live a healthy life (OECD, 2018; CIA World Factbook, 2018; WHO, n.d.). A huge chunk of the population might not live this long due to chronic diseases or other life-changing events that shorten the course of their lives.

Medicare Part D was established to serve the needs of individuals who are eligible for Parts A and B and some insurance companies offer subsidies for low-income individuals. Under federal guideline for Medicare, Part D was established in 2006 for ambulatory prescriptions (Kaiser Family Foundation, 2017). Since the inception of Part D, nearly 59 million Medicare beneficiaries have this option, if approved, to cover the cost of their prescription drugs through an individual insurance plan.

When an individual is approved for Medicare Parts A and B, it is strongly recommended that they apply for Part D during open enrollment, spanning from the 15th of October to the 7th of December each year. The costs of drugs is too high in the United States, and depending on the needs of the patient, most patients cannot afford their medication.

As chronicled by the Kaiser Family Foundation (2017), a consumer has the choice to decide between stand-alone prescription drugs plans (PDPs) or Medicare Advantage prescription drug plans. It is recommended to not sign for any plan or change plans if you do not understand any of these scenarios. If beneficiaries decide to change plans, it would save time to speak with a certified counselor who has expertise in this area. An estimated 43 million of 60 million Medicare beneficiaries are using Part D drug prescription plans (Cubanski, Damico, & Newman, 2018). The low-income subsidy program provides assistance for nearly 12 million beneficiaries in premium and cost-sharing assistance. Three firms—UnitedHealth, Humana, and CVS Health—held the biggest market share in 2018 Medicare Part D, Stand-alone PDP, and Medicare Advantage prescription drug plans, providing 55% of prescription drugs to enrollees. Medicare Part D premiums across firms differed slightly in 2018: some offered low premiums, other high. For instance, the monthly premium for PDP Humana Wal-Mart Rx was about $20 whereas it was $84 for the American Association of Retired Persons. Cost sharing for generic and brands were charged according to the tiers of the drugs. Specialty tier drugs are particularly costly (Cubanski et al., 2018).

Part D beneficiaries with PDP could pay on a sliding scale from $1 for generic drugs to $37 for branded drugs (Cubanski et al., 2018). This could be problematic for Part D holders because competition among insurance companies is pronounced. The demand for Part D will continue to rise as the population ages. This increase in demand among consumers will open doors for insurance companies to charge more, as they deem it necessary, with implicit government regulatory protocols. These insurance companies determine how much patients pay for premiums, coinsurance, and deductibles. As a consumer, your fate is determined by these providers. If consumers opt out of choosing any of the options from these providers, they will have to pay high prices out of pocket. If the government is serious about the health of its population, especially aging populations, firms providing prescriptions for senior should be regulated. If poorly regulated, competition among insurance companies will increase the cost of in-network drugs at the expense of patients. For instance, Figure 17 shows details on firms that are competing for Medicare Part D.

Figure 17: Firms competing for Medicare Part D

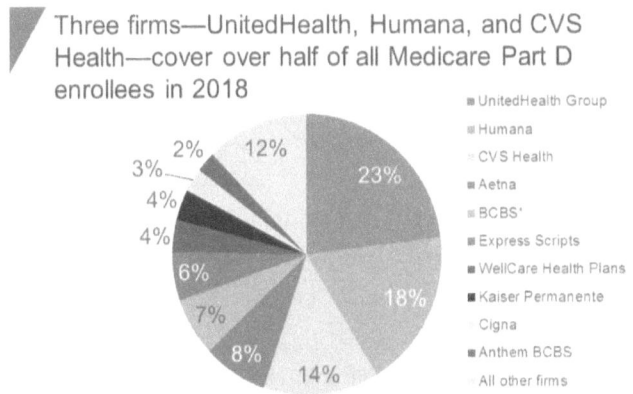

The term low-income subsidy in the U.S. healthcare system frustrates many low-income families. Depending on the state of residency and one's medical condition, subsidy programs might offer some assistance but are not sustainable and do not provide a clear strategy for patients with chronic medical conditions. Before patients can be eligible for these subsidies, they have to meet certain criteria and fill out lengthy paperwork that frustrates many. If these requirements are not met on an annual basis, patients might not receive care or, if they receive care, will be billed to pay for the cost of service. Considering that most patients requiring these subsidies have low incomes, this format affects and disrupts their care, creating a barrier for the patient. Pharmaceutical firms, local health departments, and insurance companies like subsidies to support the success of their businesses.

National Health Expenditures (NHE)

The NHE annual budget is estimated at $3.6 trillion and is expected to grow. A key component of the NHE is the personal health expenditure. The personal health expenditure has emerged to be a core driver of the high cost of U.S. healthcare. The epidemiological changes that occurred in the United States at the end of the 20th century and the beginning of the 21st century brought in another challenge. Through the 1800s and 1900s, as the population shifted from rural to urban, an unprecedented surge of infectious disease was frequent (Maeda, 2018). As public health interventions began to emerge and as those who survived the outbreak of infections aged, a dynamic shift took place from infectious to chronic diseases. Although public health interventions made significant gains to control the spread of infectious and communicative diseases, chronic diseases have become a significant threat to most Americans' lives. The advent of chronic diseases has been an underlying cause of the high cost of personal health spending on healthcare.

Official records indicate that from 1996 through 2013, personal spending on chronic disease has continued to increase without any sign of abating (Dieleman, Baral, Birger et al,.2016). Dieleman and colleagues conducted research using 183 data sources on the healthcare costs of 155 chronic medical conditions in the United States. According to the research, from 1996 to 2013, nearly $30.1 trillion was used to treat 155 medical conditions. The researchers found that diabetes was the most expensive chronic condition to treat in the healthcare system, appropriating $101.4 billion in 2013 including pharmaceutical and ambulatory care expenses. The researchers stated that ischemic heart disease was followed by diabetes, accounting for $88.1 billion, and low back and neck pain in third position accounting for $87.6 billion in 2013. The authors suggested that in 2013, personal health spending was roughly 89.5% of the U.S. NHE budget. Disease comorbidity is a driving force to increased healthcare expenditures. In 2013, cardiovascular disease had the highest personal healthcare spending with roughly $231.1 billion in the ischemic-heart-disease category. Of this expenditure, 57.3% was inpatient care whereas 65.2% went to patients 65 years and older. Further, healthcare spending was high among those aged 50 to 74 and eventually declined due to age-related mortality. Only a small portion was used by those aged 20 and younger. Spending is more for women than men. Annual healthcare spending grew by 6.4% for emergency care and 5.6%

for prescribed retail pharmaceuticals from 1996 to 2013. As discussed, the risk of these chronic diseases includes diabetes, ischemic heart disease, and chronic obstructive pulmonary disease which is a cerebrovascular disease that can be modified. Although the costs of treating chronic diseases are rising, from 1990 through 2013 spending on prescribed retail pharmaceutical care increased to $324.9 billion and $259.2 billion for emergency care in the same year (Dieleman, Baral, Birger et al, 2016).

Hospital emergency-room care does not have an established cost in the United States. Emergency-room services in the United States are set by the healthcare facility. Some might charge on a sliding scale whereas others might be quite costly. Emergency-room services cost approximately 5 to 6% of NHE but could be as high as 10% (Lee, Schuur, & Zink, 2013). The National Priorities Partnership has put forward that the emergency department could result in wasteful spending of $38 billion a year. Although emergency services in the United States are expensive, and states and private insurance companies are taking steps to reduce the cost of these services, their actions have been opposed by the American College of Emergency Physicians. Although many sources have forecasted the cost of emergency-room visits, Lee et al. (2013) recommended the Agency for Healthcare Research and Quality Medical Expenditure Panel Survey be reliable for cost forecasts. Other sources involved in the cost of emergency care are the National Hospital Ambulatory Medical Care Survey and the National Emergency Department Sample. Studies showed a discrepancy in marginal and average costs for emergency-department visits. One study showed the marginal and average cost for emergency-department visits was $88 to $209 in 1991 and $150 to $357 in 2010 (Lee et al., 2013). Another study showed that the marginal cost of outpatient emergency-department visits was $295 to $412 in 1998 and $391 to $546 in 2010. Another group of researchers found the marginal cost to be $638 in 2010. Studies on emergency-department costs are incomplete because they often use Medicare cost reports. Lee et al. used activity-based cost accounting to analyze their findings, chronicling that emergency medicine accounts for 28% of all acute care visits—roughly 130 million visits a year—and are responsible for half of all admissions.

In spite of much research on access to healthcare, few have highlighted the cost of emergency care. Lee et al. (2013) used an activity-based cost-accounting system to refute the assumption that emergency costs take up 5–6% of the NHE. The researchers built their finding on data from the Agency for Healthcare Research, Quality Medical Expenditure Panel Survey, the National Hospital Ambulatory Medical Care Survey, and the National Emergency Department Sample to conclude that the cost of emergency services could be around 6.2–10% of the NHE. In a similar vein, several studies indicated the marginal and average costs for emergency services was not uniform across medical facilities. One study reported $295 of marginal costs for outpatient emergency-department visits, $412 for an average cost in 1998, and $391 to $546 for a marginal and average cost in Michigan in 2010. In contrast, a marginal cost of $638 was reported in California hospital in 2010.

Insurance Company

Health insurance, private, commercial, and government-sponsored programs (Medicare, Medicaid, Children Health Insurance) play a vital role in the U.S. healthcare system. Insurance companies drive healthcare market costs that could become unbearable and unaffordable in the future for so many Americans. Insurance has terms that lay people might not understand when they sign up for insurance. At the onset of the Great Depression, the insurance system began to emerge in the United States to address healthcare at the demand of physicians who were concerned about patients' inability to pay for services. Insurance companies in the United States use terms like deductible, coinsurance, premiums, in-network, and tier drugs, to name a few. Most patients do not understand these terms, yet they have insurance. It is worthwhile for patients to check the insurance claim for each doctor visit. A worse scenario would be not having any insurance as some medical facility charge patients. The adoption of the ACA organized these insurances in a single place in the market to make it easy for patients to select their carrier. Regardless of which insurance company people choose, they must pay premiums and deductible charges.

The Quality of Patient Care in U.S. Fee-For-Service Versus Universal Healthcare

According to the WHO 2000 World Health Report, *Health Systems: Improving Performance,* the health system is "all the activities whose primary purpose is to promote, restore, or maintain health." A health system comprises of all "organizations, people, and actions whose primary intent is to promote, restore, or maintain health" (Fried & Gaydos, 2002, p. 29). As stated in the World Health Report 2000, the primary objectives of the healthcare system should be central to optimal health outcomes, structuring financial capacity against catastrophic payments to meet population expectations (Fried & Gaydos, 2002p.30). On this premise, health systems should provide adequate and accessible care for a population while ensuring their financial circumstances do not exclude them from seeking healthcare.

Although several studies have shed light on patients' satisfaction and experiences, a limited body of literature exists on the quality of patient care in health and global health system. The primary objective of this section is to address the effect of an entrepreneurial market-based insurance system (EHS) rather than a universal healthcare system on the quality of patient care. The question is whether EHS is cost effective in population health compared to universal access (compulsory) to obtain care in most western European states. As cited by the Institute of Medicine and Committee on Quality of Health Care in America (2001), the provision of health services should be based on safety, effectiveness, patient-centeredness, timeliness, efficiency, and equitable care (Fried & Gaydos, 2002, p. 33). However, the entrepreneurial model of healthcare delivery in the United States has undeniably been delivered through biomedical intervention with limited access to a holistic population-based approach that is accessible and affordable by all. This market-based model in the U.S. health system has created inequity and inequality to health, manifested in patient–provider relationships.

The fee-for-service model of healthcare delivery adopted by the United States over half a century ago has clearly left an unprecedented mark because of undistributed access to care, prejudice, lack of affordability, demographic and geographic composition, and geopolitical influence. This fee-for-service model contrasts with the compulsory health system in the United Kingdom (UK), Canada, Japan, Israel, and most western European countries, where tax revenues fund healthcare and everyone gets a fair share through universal coverage (Donaldson & Bryan, 2012). The entrepreneur model is substantially privatized and voluntary in the United States. It does not contain costs and access to care becomes unevenly distributed. Those who are sicker become vulnerable to care access, and in most cases, patients' evaluations rest on their socioeconomic status (Arpey, Gaglioti, & Rosenbaum, 2017). The evaluation of the patient–provider relationship in recent time has become an integrated part of the health system. Most medical facilities in the health system are now regulated based on patient satisfaction and experience. Patient satisfaction correlates with patient care and hence, clinical outcome (Chen, Zou, Shuster, 2017).

The quality of patient care through an affordable service in the current state of the U.S. healthcare system remains uncertain. The U.S. entrepreneurial healthcare model addresses population health through biomedical intervention and market-based insurance schemes that are costly (Donaldson & Bryan, 2012). The absence of the central government in the mainstream health-system domain has accompanied an imbalance in competition among private national insurance companies (Donaldson & Bryan, 2012).

From their view, "plus choice," when everyone has coverage with the choice to add private insurance, is seen to be a more conciliatory approach to the U.S. healthcare dilemma. The adoption of a single-payer healthcare system intervention in the U.S. state of Vermont, for example, could save the state up to 25% on healthcare expenditures in 10 years; much more cost effective than ACA reform in 2010. Furthermore, the implementation of Medicare, Medicaid, and the Veteran's Administration under U.S. entrepreneurial health delivery is indicative that a compulsory comprehensive health system could be effective for patient-centered care and contain costs (Donaldson & Bryan, 2012).

The integrated component of quality patient care has not been fully adopted in the U.S. EHS model of public health. The problem with this economic model of healthcare is that resources are inappropriately allocated (Kinder, & Isham, 2014). The population health model adopted by the University of Wisconsin suggests that social and economic factors (40%) substantially affect health outcome. In contrast, clinical activity impacts only 20% of the U.S. population's health outcomes. In the United States, 25% of monetary resources allocated to health services are deemed ineffective (Kindig & Isham, 2014).

Central to the core of population health are perceived perceptions, socioeconomic status, barriers to care, cost of care, and physician burnout, all inadequately addressed in the EHS model of care. The provider–patient relationship can affect the quality of patient care (Arpey, Gaglioti, and Rosenbaum, 2017). Socioeconomic status can be a factor in care. In the entrepreneurial model of the health system, perceptions of clinicians on patients' socioeconomic status has a direct effect on healthcare delivery and use (Arpey et al., 2017).

The Significance of Quality Patient Care in the Health System

Although it has been found in several studies the importance of patient satisfaction and patient-centeredness in the health system, a few has supported the rationale of quality patient care in EHS. The patient–provider relationship has emerged over the years to be a significant driver of population health, and consequentially, the healthcare system. This section will add to the body of literature that examines the quality of patient care in the global health system. Although the EHS model in the United States has proven effective in biomedical intervention, it has been costly and less effective in addressing population health from a holistic perspective through the lens of patient-centered care.

The epidemiological transition that occurred in the United States nearly a hundred years ago has left the society with another problem. A transition from infectious disease to chronic and degenerative disease has led to longevity (Fried & Gaydos, 2002, p.12). The third epidemiological transition has been a reemergence of infectious disease on the global stage as a result of exchanges in social, demographic, and environmental public health challenges; technological evolution; and international commercialization (Fried & Gaydos, 2002, p. 13). Chronic and degenerative diseases have taken a consistent toll on the population, altering the course of mortality, morbidity, and disability that has transformed international health systems. A report from

CDC (2015) suggested that the ten leading causes of death in the United States are heart disease (635,260); cancer (598,038); accidents/unintentional injuries (161,374); chronic lower respiratory disease (154,596); stroke (cerebrovascular diseases—142,142); Alzheimer's disease (116,103); diabetes (80,058); influenza and pneumonia (51, 537); nephritis, nephrotic syndrome, and nephrosis (50,046); and international self-harm (suicide: 44,965). The number of deaths reported per 100,000 populations in 2015 was 844, with the infant mortality rate at 5.9 per 1,000 live births. The average life expectancy in the United States is 78.8 years. The course of disease in the U.S. population disproportionally affects those of particular races and ethnicities, according to the level of access, care, and support.

Although heart disease is the leading cause of death in the United States, it disproportionally affects Black people. The rate of heart disease among Blacks or African Americans was 210 per 100,000 population in 2015 compared with 171.9 in White people at the national level (CDC, n.d.). Access to primary and maternal care has influenced infant mortality. Under-five-year-old children born to Black people per 100, 000 are 10.9 times more likely to die compared to 4.9 in Whites, 5 in Hispanics, and 7.7 in American Indians. In the United States, the burden of disease risk factor underscores primary population health interventions. An estimated 17% of the U.S. adult populations uses tobacco product while 11% of the youth population smokes (CDC, 2015). In 2016, nearly 30% of the U.S. adult population was obese, and 14% of youth in 2015. HIV affects an estimated 17% of the U.S. population. In a similar manner,

Hepatitis B cases are nearly 1.1% and hepatitis C prevalence is 0.80% in the national population (CDC, 2015). Although vaccinations have proven to reduce the risk of preventable diseases, national influenza-vaccine coverage in the United States in 2016 was only 47%. In 2015, child vaccination covered nearly 72% of the national population. Even though screening in primary health systems could increase the rate of detecting preventable or treatable diseases at early onset, an estimated 69% of the U.S. population had colorectal cancer screening in 2014 (CDC, n.d.).

Despite making significant gains in lifespan through public health initiatives, the impact of epidemiological and demographical transitions has not only affected the population on the individual level but on the national level as well. At the national level (macro level) or local (micro level) institutional levels, healthcare policy should be clearly conceptualized in ways that are cost effective, high quality, serviceable, accessible, technologically friendly, affordable, marketed, and regulated to a level that fosters nurturing and mutually binding relationships between patients and healthcare providers, particularly in populations that are classified as vulnerable and at risk of financial hardship. Low socioeconomic can affect longevity, quality of life, and is a risk factor for chronic disease (Kindig & Isham, 2014). Those in the category of low socioeconomic status, when compared with those with high socioeconomic status, are less likely to have integrated access to care, due to high costs. Those with low socioeconomic status are often perceived by physicians as less intelligent, irresponsible, and dependent on the system, and might be perceived to be less likely to comply with medical advice (Kindig & Isham, 2014). In contrast to this perception, Gulliford et al. (2002) argued that access to care means to coordinate or make resources available for consumers to use and improve their health. Access could be impacted by financial, organizational, and social barriers. If these barriers are removed, it could smooth the use of healthcare services (Gulliford et al., 2002). In a similar vein Downing, Bates, and Longhurst (2018) chronicled that the alarming number of physicians leaving the healthcare workforce due to burnout should be concerning to the future of the medical field and can affect patient care and the health system.

The U.S. EHS model has sometimes worked but has also sometimes failed. The national health expenditure has reached nearly $3.6 trillion (CMS, 2018; World Bank, 2018; CIA World Factbook, 2018; & WHO, n.d.). The United States has the highest GDP (18%) for healthcare and per capita ($10,109) among industrialized nations in the world (International Monetary Fund, 2018). Although healthcare financing plays a key role in the health system, its correlation to population health outcomes should be explored. Despite spending so much on healthcare, the U.S. approach to population health remains highly contested. Statistics from CDC (2018) show that 86% of the U.S. $2.7 trillion monetary resources allocated on healthcare expenditures are specifically for individuals with chronic medical conditions or some form of mental illness. Among other chronic diseases that affect the U.S. population and thus the healthcare system are heart disease and stroke, cancer, diabetes, obesity, arthritis, Alzheimer's disease, epilepsy, tooth decay, and risk factors that include sedentary lifestyle and excessive alcohol consumption.

The impact of heart disease and stroke is costly to the U.S. economy. The economic burden to the health system costs nearly $190 billion a year. The annual to lost productivity and decrease in job viability is expected to exceed $126 billion (CDC, 2018). Nearly 810,000 Americans die from heart disease or stroke every year. Statistics from the CDC (2018) suggest that the annual incidence of cancer in the United States is 1.7 million with 600,000 experiencing mortality. Cancer has been the second leading cause of mortality after heart disease in the United States for the past few years. The economic burden of cancer on the U.S. health system has been projected to be $174 billion by 2020. Even more prevalent in the U.S. population is diabetes. More than 29 million Americans have diabetes and 86 million are prediabetic. The annual cost for treating diabetes alone costs the U.S. health system $245 billion per year (CDC, 2018)

One in 5 U.S. children and 1 in 3 U.S. adults are obese. The economic cost of obesity on this EHS costs $147 billion each year. In a similar way, arthritis takes a heavy toll on nearly 54.4 million U.S. adults (CDC, 2018). This chronic pain is the number one leading cause of work-related disability in the United States. In 2013, treating arthritis alone cost the U.S. health system $304 billion, and nearly $140 billion was allocated to direct medical costs while $164 billion went to indirect costs and related lost earnings. An estimated 5.7 million Americans are affected by Alzheimer's disease, cited as the six-leading cause of death (CDC, 2018). In 2010, the cost of treating Alzheimer's disease increased from $159 billion to $215 billion. Alzheimer's disease treatment is expected to cost between $379 billion and $500 billion a year by 2040. In the United States, epilepsy affects

3 million adults and 470,000 children and teens. The cost of epilepsy is an annual $15.5 billion in the U.S. EHS.

U.S. EHS institutions are operated by private, public, and federal and local government entities. The system has multiple layers; it is at an individual state's discretion to regulate insurance companies. Failure on the part of the state to regulate the already complicated insurance scheme can create financial catastrophic for patients. A major component of the health system should be to improve the health status of its population (Fried & Gaydos, 2002). The health system should aim to protect citizens from the pitfalls of financial hardship that could be caused by health-related expenses (Fried & Gaydos, 2002, p. 36). A sustainable health system should not create financial crisis or hardship for those who seek care. An optimal healthcare financing system should include a revenue-generating system that could provide care for people without exposing them to risk factors such as poverty (Fried & Gaydos, 2002). Individuals should have access to care through public or private services. According to the WHO (2007) framework, healthcare financing 1) should have adequate funds for effective use of healthcare financing, 2) out-of-pocket spending should be alternated with prepaid insurances schemes like insurance risk pooling, 3) the poor should have access to finances mitigating financial hardship that directly results from health cost, 4) the system should be evaluated to maintain efficient use of resources, 5) financial system should be transparent through information sharing, and 6) information should be readily available on health system financing (Fried & Gaydos, 2002, p. 36)

In the United States, the degree to which insurance companies operate and coordinate remains questionable. In 2016 an estimated 49% of the U.S. national population had employer-based insurance (Kff.org, 2016). Of the population, 19% had healthcare coverage through Medicaid, 14% through Medicare, 2% public, 7% non-group, and 9% of the general population had no coverage. Aligned with federal guidelines, those with incomes below 100% of the federal poverty level among nonelderly younger than 64 years received nearly 55% of a Medicaid-based insurance benefit in 2016. Approximately 18% were uninsured, 14% had employer-based insurance, 4% public, and 9% non-group insurance (Kff.org, 2016). Although the landmark 2010 ACA legislation brought the U.S. health system closer to universal access to care, parallel to the mandatory system in many western European nations, it has not been fully implemented. Statistics from Kff.org (2016) implied that 15% of children aged 0–18 did not have access to insurance, coupled with 85% of nonelderly adults between the ages of 19 and 64. These statistics acknowledged the implication of the U.S. health system that fails to provide access to care to undocumented immigrants who might be caught in the middle of the healthcare debate. Although working-class and middle-class income groups are major contributors to the U.S. economy, uneven access to care raises a significant question about the U.S. healthcare model of care. In 2016, 75% of at least full-time workers had no access to insurance while 11% of part-time workers fit in the same category. According to Kff.org (2016), nearly 44% of nonelderly Whites had no source of insurance, similar to 33% of Hispanics, and 15% of Blacks.

The epidemiological health profile of the U.S. population requires a compulsory comprehensive health system to address the need of it growing demand from chronic disease. Such a system would require a sustainable relationship between stakeholders to optimize and operationalize a health system that would be cost effective. The quality of patient care through an affordable care system in the current state of U.S. healthcare remains uncertain. Unlike universal coverage in Canada and most European countries, where single payer is used, the U.S. EHS model addresses population health through multiple layers and market-based insurance schemes that are costly and, at times, uncoordinated. The problem with this economic model of healthcare system is that resources are not allocated to the right purpose (Kindig & Isham, 2014).

Stakeholders

The quality of care has emerged as a significant factor on the quality of healthcare in population health. Although several researchers studied patient satisfaction, patient-centeredness, and patient experiences (Chen, Zou, & Shuster, 2017), a limited number described the impact of patient–provider relationships on the quality of patient care. Key stakeholders are not limited to federal, state, and local governments; patients; communities; macro and microinsurance insurance companies; healthcare professionals; and international nongovernmental organizations (vital in the developing world) in the healthcare systems.

As the U.S. population ages, increases in size, and decreases in growth and fertility rate (1.80), it could be significant to invest in population health. Currently, the 329.7 million population has a growth rate of 0.7%, the GDP per capita in the United States corresponds to $59,774 with a projected growth rate of 2.8% (OECD, 2008). The United States has a 10.5% of GDP tax on personal income. The unemployment rate in the U.S. labor force is estimated at 4.4% with the government accounting for 136.3% of GDP. The United States is one of the most unequal industrialized countries in the world, accounting for a 0.39 Gini coefficient compared to 0.29 for France. In 2016, the United States had a total poverty ratio of about 0.178 in comparison to 0.081 in France and 0.142 in Canada (OECD, 2018).

The United States spends far more than any other developed nation on healthcare. The health spending per capita in 2017 reached $10,209 in contrast to $4,264 in the United Kingdom. Voluntary spending on private insurance per capita of GDP in the UK was $900.00 in contrast to $1,785 in the United States. Government compulsory spending per capita in the United States for Medicare, for example, was nearly $8,047, compared to $3,341 in the UK.

The population health model dictates the progressive participation of healthcare professionals. Increases to access to care address some of the most pressing needs of patients. In contrast, limited access to care creates a worsening environment and poor state of health. The United States has geographical variation in physicians who serve in primary care. Rural areas are asymmetrically affected in the distribution of healthcare providers. In 2017, the United States had 2.6 physicians for 1,000 people in contrast to 4.2

per 1,000 in Germany and 5.1 in Austria (OECD, 2018). In contrast to 17.7 nurses per 1,000 inhabitants in Norway, the United States had 11.6 nurses per 1,000 populations and the UK had 7.9 in 2017. As to the number of hospital beds, the United States had 2.8 per 1,000 people in 2017 and the total length of hospital stay was 5.50 days (OECD, 2018).

Although healthcare systems around the world have evolved to influence population health, the U.S. EHS approach has been ineffective to coordinate and improve population health in comparison to the National Health Service (NHS) in England (Seervai, Shah, & Osborn, 2017) and social health insurance in Germany, France, Israel, Belgium, The Netherlands, Japan, and Switzerland (Fried, & Gaydos, 2012, p. 55). Although the U.S. healthcare system is considered one of the most technologically advanced healthcare infrastructures in the world, it has failed to ensure universal access to its population (Fried & Gaydos, 2012, p.963). Universal coverage, where everyone gets fair share with the choice to add private insurance has shown to be effective in national health services in the UK and other European countries. Most countries with universal access to care have a single-payer system through government and employer-finances insurance run through insurance companies.

Although the landmark ACA legislation of 2010 drew the U.S. healthcare system closer to universal care, it was rife with legal battles (Donaldson & Bryan, 2012). The ACA provided coverage to nearly 32 million Americans and protected patients' right to coverage on preexisting conditions. Although ACA was groundbreaking in U.S. history, its legality and constitutionality to compel individuals to purchase insurance was challenged in the judiciary system. Opponents of the ACA argued that it could cost taxpayers more while proponents contended the benefit would outweigh the cost (Donaldson & Bryan, 2012).

In contrast to EHS, social health insurance (SHI) implemented in Germany, France, Israel, Belgium, The Netherlands, Japan, Switzerland, and some Latin and Central American countries is delivered by mandatory mechanisms through quasiprivate insurers or social insurers (Fried & Gaydos, 2002, p. 54). This system is financed by payroll tax deductions and supplemented with tax revenue. Employers and employees share the cost. The source of financing SHI might also include donations from internal charitable organizations that could be a bilateral or multilateral aid. The SHI model, particularly in Germany, has been cost effective through sickfunds that prevent workers from financial catastrophic due to medical expenses.

The concept of population health is rooted in understanding the advent of chronic and acute disease such as obesity, addiction, mental health, and the reemergence of infectious diseases (Kayes & Galea, 2016; Oleske, 2009; Mesesan Schmitz, 2015). Collective effort is needed to build a public-health intervention for population health (Kayes & Galea, 2016). Keen on the core value of population health, Kayes and Galea (2016) suggested the advance of technological innovation in the healthcare infrastructure has become instrumental in the 21st century to understand the nature of disease. Although Mesesan (2015) and Kindig and Isham (2014) supported the authors' argument that population health should benefit all, the conceptual framework is yet to be implemented in U.S. healthcare reform where collective effort is perceived to be a socialist notion. Integration of population health in hospitals expands on the care of patients (Morrison, 2014). Population health is inclusive—medical and nonmedical—and has not been the focus of the health system. However, this narrative continues to shift as hospitals provide integrated care (Morrison, 2014).

Review of Studies and the Impact of U.S. Healthcare

Three types of insurance systems exist in Europe that are crucially important for universal coverage (Seervai, Shah, & Osborn, 2017): those dominated by public insurance, regulated private insurance, and mixed public–private insurance. Critical analysis of insurance systems led to universal adoption in most European countries. System implementations might be limited in countries that lack welfare or social-policy systems. Low GDP economies where government bureaucracies are unstructured and sometimes inefficient in collecting taxes could find it difficult to contrive these insurance systems. Governments use tax revenues to fund the health system and lack of tax revenues could incapacitate governments in low GDP countries to provide universal coverage to provide for the welfare of their populations.

Universal coverage provides access to healthcare for every resident. The state provides essential health services and everyone has access to healthcare, regardless of their ability to pay (The Commonwealth Fund. n.d.; Seervai,

Shah, & Osborn, 2017). Most countries with universal access to care have single-payer systems financed through government and employer insurance system. Countries universally adopt public insurance schemes and their finance and delivery methods are operated through a single-payer system. Governments use tax revenues to fund public insurance. Care is delivered through government contracts or direct work with providers. A common example exists in the English NHS. This system provides coverage for every resident. Although the NHS is comprehensive, it does not cover mental healthcare and dental but has some coverage for eye care. The NHS system does not require copayment during service. An estimated 10% of UK residents have a limited amount of coverage through private insurance provided by employers because all citizens are entitled to state-funded access to care (The Commonwealth Fund. n.d.; Seervai et al., 2017).

Regulated private insurance is a form of universal access to care financed through private insurance regulated by governments (Seervai et al., 2017). A model of this system exists in The Netherlands. Insurance companies in this system operate on competition but are nonprofit entities that allow individuals choice of insurance. Employer–employee pooling systems are redistributed to insurers according to risk factors to minimize the risk of picking only healthy enrollees. Private providers who provide services to the population according to their needs are then reimbursed by insurance companies: a system similar to the Medicare reimbursement process. In The Netherlands, it is mandatory for all residents to purchase insurance except when exempted. In most cases, those who are underprivileged or in the low-income category receive a subsidy from government funds to compensate for premium payments, similar to Medicaid in the United States. It is at the government's discretion to determine the insurance package. Consumers are charged deductibles or out-of-pocket expenses. In contrast, services that include primary care, maternity care, home nursing care, and care for children are deductible-free. Like the UK system, the Dutch system allows people to add private insurance.

In mixed public–private insurance, the system combines public and private enterprise financing (Seervai et al., 2017). A good example can be found in France. In the French system, taxes are the financing source for nonprofit health insurance funds. The central government uses tax revenues to fund health-insurance delivery through nonprofit organizations. The government regulates, supersedes, and negotiates funds in the insurance system. Identical to the UK and The Netherlands, residents have the choice to add private insurance, and like the U.S. ACA, patients choose their insurance in the marketplace. It is also mandatory in this system for all residents to access healthcare funded by the state. In contrast to the United States, where most individuals pay for their insurance through employer-sponsor programs, in a mixed insurance system, diagnostic tests coupled with prescription drugs can be covered. Dissimilar to the U.S. EHS, mixed systems include cost sharing for a doctor visit, inpatient stay, and dental and vision services. In France's mixed insurance system, out-of-pocket expenditures cover private insurance subsidized by the government, like Medigap supplemental insurance in the United States. As suggested, universal coverage as part of the ACA is already in effect in the states of Massachusetts, California, and Minnesota (Seervai et al., 2017).

According to The Commonwealth Fund (n.d.), the U.S. EHS provides healthcare services that are distinct from those of the UK, France, Canada, and The Netherlands. In the U.S. healthcare system, each individual state has a pivotal role in regulating private insurance. Private or employer-based insurances are payroll deductions. State and private insurance are crucial in the U.S. EHS entrepreneur system. In 2015, nearly 67.2% of the U.S. population had coverage through private voluntary health insurance. Nearly 56% had employer-sponsored programs compared to 15% with direct coverage. Publicly funded programs provided access to nearly 37% of the population. In contrast to the United States, private health insurance does not comprise a significant proportion of the UK health system. In 2015, about 10.5% of the UK population had private health insurance. Unlike the complex nature of navigating the private-insurance system in the United States, UK private health insurance provides convenient access to care. However, the majority of policies in the UK have no plan for mental health, maternity services, emergency, and general practice. The U.S. ACA mandates essential health services and that private insurance companies carry these services. Limited data is available on private insurance in the UK (The Commonwealth Fund, n.d.).

Although the U.S. healthcare system might differ from most universal coverage policies, arguably it offers mixed public insurance similar to France and the UK. U.S. Medicare, Medicaid, and CHIP provide affordable care for seniors and low-income families. Medicare plays a vital role in the U.S. health system, reimbursing coverage for hospitalization, physician services, prescription drugs, and supplementary programs. Medicare programs can also be used to eliminate the cost sharing intended for preventive services (The Commonwealth Fund, n.d.). Medicare could be traditional or Advantage. Traditional Medicare beneficiaries use open networks based on fee-for-service whereas Advantage is subsidized by the federal government through a private insurer, based on the network plan. The downside of Medicare is that it does not cover long-term care but only postacute care. In contrast, Medicaid offers coverage for long-term care.

The U.S. health system is 49% publicly financed and consumes 18% of GDP. In contrast, The Commonwealth Fund (n.d.) noted that in 2014 the UK allocated 9.9% or 10% of its GDP to healthcare. The NHS accounted for 79.5% of healthcare expenditure and is publicly financed. Taxation is the main source of UK public healthcare financing whereas a limited amount comes from national insurance (payroll deductions similar to the United States). Patients who which to use NHS as a private insurer are obliged to make certain copays that could be part of NHE revenue. In the United States, Medicare can be financed through payroll deductions or taxes, premiums, and government revenues. Although states oversee Medicaid, it is tax-funded with federal oversight. Funds for Medicaid from federal to state governments are matching funds with substantial rate differentials per capita that could range from 50% to 74% (The Commonwealth Fund, n.d.). The federal government funds Medicaid expansion under the ACA. As of 2014, private insurance comprised 39% of U.S. NHE. Private insurance could be for-profit and nonprofit and receive oversight from state insurance commissioners, who are subject to federal regulations (The Commonwealth Fund, n.d.). However, the degree to which these regulatory policies are implemented remains questionable with thousands of micro- and macroinsurances in the market system. It is the individual's prerogative to buy private insurance, which can be funded through voluntary, tax-exempt premiums with cost sharing between employees and employers on the employers' terms. The employer tax exemption comprises the third largest U.S. healthcare expenditure after Medicare and Medicaid; an exemption that has reduced government revenue by $260 billion per year (The commonwealth Fund, n.d.).

Although health systems around the world, particularly in high GDP economies, strive to improve patient care and transparency in healthcare organizations, the U.S. EHS model began contemplating the EHR system in 2005. The EHR health-information technology surfaced with the enactment of the 2009 American Recovery and Reinvestment Act, which cost about $30 million investment (The Commonwealth Fund, n.d.). The system was put in place to reward hospitals and physicians that use EHR systems. In 2014 an estimated 84% of U.S. physicians had mastery of some kind of EHR, which has seen an eightfold increase since 2008 (The Commonwealth Fund, n.d.). The program focuses on information exchange. In contrast, 98% of primary care physician have used EHR in the UK since the advent of the system. Although EHR and information technology have galvanized health systems in high-income countries, use in the EHS has caused debate over cost and benefit in patient care. Although EHR has increased data transparency, some researchers have argued that the skyrocketing costs in personal health expenditures in the U.S. health system could have a negative impact on patients.

As implied by Echouffo-Tcheugui, Bishu, Fonarow, Egede (2017), The U.S. EHS has fostered a health system that has not been patient-centered or population minded, beginning with the adoption of Medicare in the 1960s. The cost of personal care has increased over time. The epidemiological transition has led to increased degenerative chronic diseases like cancer, heart disease, and obesity. In contrast, the demographical transition created urban flight a century ago. In recent years, White flight created inner-city occupation by a majority low-income population where access to clinical services is sometimes illusory. In a similar vein, many rural areas are in dire need of healthcare facilities.

Although health systems in high-income countries are entranced with the use of technology and EHR (Lowery, 2012), it could take years for low GDP countries with less than $1,000 Gini per capita to catch up. EHR provides safety and confidentiality to not only the patient, but family members as well. Although paper-based bookkeeping might be obsolete or at a minimum in advanced countries, it is a widely accepted practice in low-income countries. The advent of the EHR has revolutionized the medical record system. Although it might be feasible to employ EHR in medical facilities, the cost associated with these advances are pricey for the healthcare organization. Although EHR could be effective in reducing medical errors and increasing work productivity, not every researcher agrees with this assessment. Some have argued that EHR and health-information technology can increase patient costs (Kumar, 2011).

Although the U.S. healthcare system has been mixed in addressing population health with a pay-for-service approach, some would argue that the intervention of EHR was a major step in reinvigorating the already-complicated system. However, Kumar (2011) disagreed with this assessment and proposed that high technology in the healthcare industry has led to high costs. Low-income GDP countries face the consequences. These countries lack the resources to finance their healthcare systems. With chronic diseases replacing infectious diseases, these countries might need low-cost technology to keep up with the growing demand of healthcare consumption, training their healthcare workers in accordance with or at least managing the standard in high GDP countries. In spite of Kumar's (2011) reservations, others are optimistic about EHR (Seymour, Frantsvog, & Graeber, 2012; DesRoches, Cambell, Rao et al., 2008). According to Seymour et al. (2012), EHR is responsible for reducing medical error, despite some resistance from the medical community to adopt the system.

Seymour et al. (2012) found that the introduction of EHR has increased hospital expenditures and high costs to maintain the functionality of the technology in the healthcare system. In spite of the mixed reaction to costs and benefits of EHR in the healthcare system, the benefits of EHR include clinical workflow, provision of credible documentation, improved data quality, collections due from patients, and the portability of data for quality assurance. The manifestation of EHR in the postmodern world has enhanced the use of effective and efficient functions, physician orders, laboratory functionality, and multifunctionality in the clinical workspace.

An increase in EHR use aligns with data quality and safety. The legislation for all healthcare providers to use EHR was established by the Bush administration in 2005. According to Seymour et al. (2012), the complex web of U.S. healthcare by many players and the need for a standardized system led to implementation of EHR. EHR includes patients' personal identifiable information and only those in direct patient care should have access to EHR. The EHR system has also enabled those in medical practice to formulate a coding system that is user specific. These specifications have been vital to determine the cost of personal health expenditures in the United States. From 1996 to 2013 nearly $30.1 trillion was used to treat 155 medical conditions (Dieleman, Baral, & Birger et al., 2016). Among these conditions, diabetes was the most expensive chronic condition to be treated in the healthcare system, appropriated $101.4 billion in 2013.

Despite this extravagant spending, the United States undoubtedly stands alone among industrialized countries lacking universal coverage. The health system in the United States has ushered in limited access to protect patients from financial hardship and access to care when needed. Ischemic heart disease, followed by diabetes, accounted for $88.1 billion of U.S. health cost in 2013 (Dieleman et al., 2016). In a similar vein, low back and neck pain accounted for virtually $87.6 billion in the same year. In 2013 personal health spending was roughly 89.5% of U.S. NHE. Disease comorbidity has become the driving cost in the healthcare system, increasing the cost of personal PHE per year. The burden of disease, disability, and associated economic cost has created a vacuum in the U.S. healthcare system. In 2013, cardiovascular disease had the highest PHE, with roughly $231.1 billion in the ischemic heart disease category. Of this expenditure, 57.3% was for inpatient services whereas 65.2% went to patients 65 years and older. According to research findings, healthcare spending was high among those aged 50 to 74 and eventually declined due to age-related mortality. Only a small mortality sample accrued for those age 20 and younger (Dieleman et al., 2016). Although these findings are objective, they are not exhaustive in explaining U.S. NHE. These few examples are in the high category of chronic diseases that consume most health funds in the United States.

Synthesis

The WHO framework on population health is narrowly been practiced not only in the EHS but also in low GDP countries that struggle to keep up with the demand of their populations. Although the objective of the health system is to protect people against financial catastrophy and ensuring every citizen has access to equitable healthcare, the market-based approach is a mixture of welfare and a national health system that inundates the system leaving many without access to care. The problem is this system is too costly and creates disparity. The EHS focuses on improving population health. In the case of the United States, the ACA, brought the country closer to universal health coverage. Whether an EHS can provide a health system that is just, accessible, fair, and evenly distributed is yet to be seen.

In contrast to the U.S. EHS structure, shown in Figure 18, which does not guarantee every American the right to care, the UK NHS structure shown in Figure 19 guaranteed every resident access to care. In a similar way, the Canadian health system, portrayed in Figure 20, was constructed on the ideological platform that healthcare was a fundamental right and not a choice. The health system built on the platform that individual need to healthcare should be addressed (Martin et al., 2018). The Canadian Medicare system, contravened in 1947, passed through several amendments to adopt federal cost sharing. Although decentralized through a provincial and territorial insurance system, it does not require a copay at the point of care. Despite these advantages of the Canadian health system, access to care has been inadequate for indigenous populations.

Figure 18 US Health System Structure

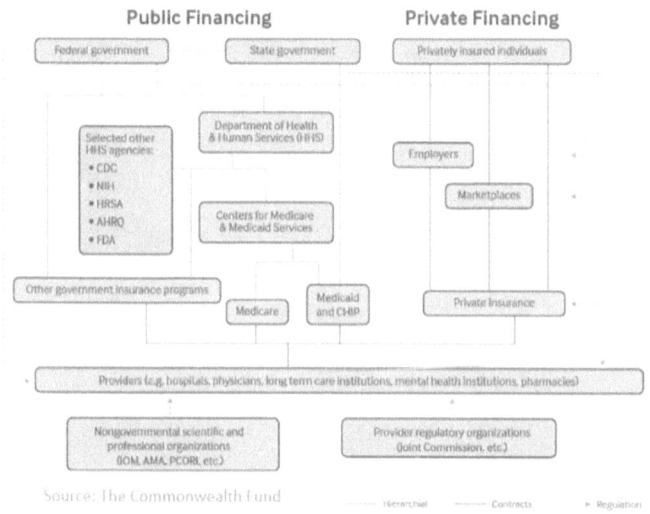

Figure 19 UK Health System structure

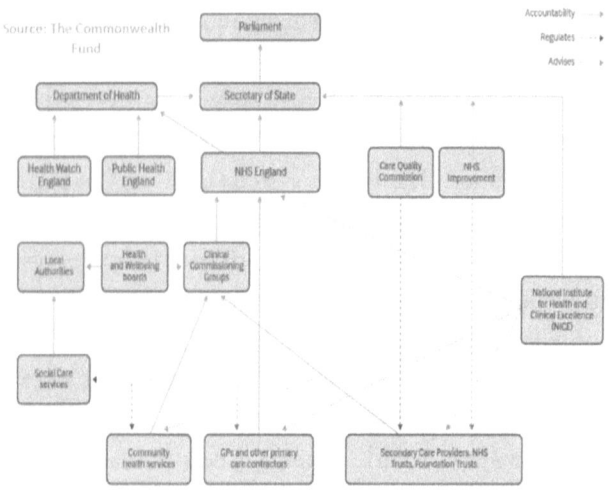

Figure 20 Canadian health-system structure

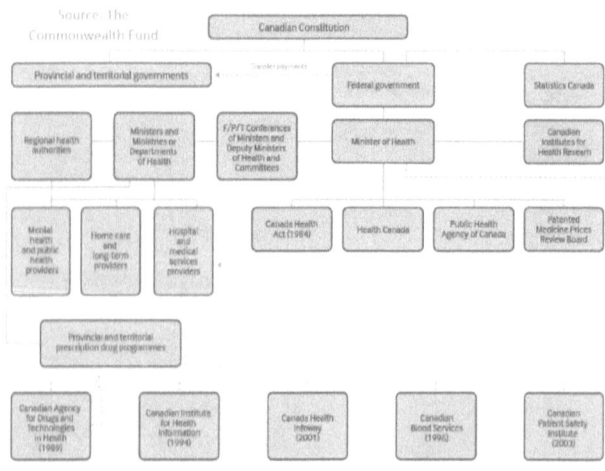

Long queues and access to care are not well coordinated for indigenous groups, raising doubts about the Canadian population health model (Martin et al., 2018). Much-needed effort from public engagement could help resolve issues or concerns of underserved populations. Although the Canadian health system is not nationalized, it does require national scrutiny. The health system is publicly funded through taxation, providing universal access to medical and hospital services for the Canadian people. In contrast to Canada's decentralized system, that upholds the fundamental principle that access to health should be provided on a need basis, the United States is the only Western country that implements unequal access to care, despite passing the ACA into law.

The difference between the two systems is that Canada sees itself as a collective population-health approach whereas the United States narrowly focus on an individual-health approach (Martin et al., 2018). Medicare in Canada is publicly funded with a single payer. For funding purposes, all three territories and the 10 provinces of Canada must adhere to a federal standard through universality, accessibility, and portability in comprehensive care. In the portability scheme, Canadian residents carry their insurance whenever they travel inside the country, which allows them to access care when needed. Universality ensures informality of insurance: all else being equal, terms and policies apply equally, which means that under no circumstances does private access overshadow national universal care. For accessibility, Canadians are not required to make payment at the time of service. Unlike in the United States, people do not pay deductibles. Canadian healthcare spending is about 10.4% of their GDP.

The quality of patient care has changed dramatically in the global health system. Although patient care remains a significant factor in the healthcare system, access to care is understudied. Health systems are not uninform: each country has its own policies and strategic frameworks that place its citizen at a tipping point in the healthcare system (Petrou, Samoutis, Lionis, 2018). One common goal, however, is the health of the population. Although it matters how healthcare organizations deliver health services, it is more critical how these services are used: that is, whether services are designed to the needs of the population, as the global community consumes healthcare in different ways. In their analysis of social health insurance in France, Germany, Israel, Luxembourg, The Netherlands, and Switzerland, Polikowski, Santos-Eggimann (2002) found that in Switzerland and Germany, healthcare delivery was more comprehensive with comparable total health expenditures. The authors implied that universal access to care in most high-GDP per capita countries was a universal practice, apart from the United States.

The national health systems in the UK or the Scandinavian and Mediterranean countries do not exclude taxpayers who have difficulty paying. All taxpayers benefit from the system. The challenge of the system, however, is the wait time to see a provider. Despite the universality of access to care, affordability is becoming more concerning as countries begin to consider out-of-pocket payment schemes. Statutory, compulsory, or entrepreneur systems might not provide individuals with all the coverage needed because people have an option to purchase additional insurance from the private market. Universal coverage might not mean unlimited care. In The Netherlands, the package of comprehensive healthcare includes necessity, effectiveness, efficiency, and individual payment. New Zealand, in contrast, uses the National Health Committee model for effectiveness, efficiency, equity, and acceptability. In Sweden, the Parliamentary Commission adopted an ethical principle centered on human dignity, need, solidarity, and cost-efficiency (Polikowski, Santos-Eggimann, 2002).

In the United States, the 2010 ACA, enacted to nationalize the health insurance system, is far from providing universal care. The U.S. EHS provides healthcare services that are distinct from those in the UK, France, Canada, and The Netherlands. In the U.S. healthcare system, the state plays a pivotal role in regulating private insurance. Private or employer-based insurances are deducted from payrolls. Both insurances are crucial in the U.S. EHS.

Although the U.S. healthcare system significantly differs from that of most universal-coverage policies, it arguably offers mixed public insurance similar to most Western European countries. U.S. Medicare, Medicaid, and CHIP provide affordable care for seniors and low-income families. Medicare plays a vital role in the U.S. health system, used to reimburse coverage for hospitalization, physician services, prescription drugs, and supplementary programs. In contrast to universal healthcare, where access to care has a single payer through government and an employer-financed insurance system that is run through insurance companies (Seervai, Shah, & Osborn, 2017), the United States has multiple payers, complicating the system for patients to navigate.

In 2015 nearly 67.2% of the U.S. population had coverage through private voluntary health insurance. Nearly 56% had employer-sponsored programs compared to 15% with direct coverage. Publicly funded programs provided access to nearly 37% of the population in a similar way to Medicare and Medicaid, 16% and 18% respectively. The percentage of direct purchase was 16% while 4.7% covers armed forces personnel. In the U.S. healthcare system, an immigrant without legal status is ineligible for health coverage; however, federally funded health facilities do not discriminate against individuals in accessing emergency services, regardless of their ability to pay at the time of service, closely aligned with the welfare system in the UK and France (The Commonwealth Fund, n.d.).

In 2015, nearly two-thirds of ineligible immigrants did not have access to basic insurance. Private insurance plays a significant role in the U.S. healthcare system. Nearly 66% of the populations are covered by an employer or individual-based insurance with supplementation to Medicare for those 65 years and older. Primary care delivery is private, consisting of mixed or nonprofit hospitals (~70% of beds), public (~15%) and for-profit (~15%). Payment for provider service has mostly been fee for service, private plans, and incentives. According to the ACA 2010 service mandate, every health plan and small business group that has more than 50 employees is mandated to provide insurance to individuals that covers ambulatory service, emergency service, hospitalization, maternal and newborn, mental health services and substance-use-disorder treatment, prescription drugs, rehabilitative services and devices, laboratory services, preventive and wellness services, chronic-disease management, pediatric services, and dental and vision care (The Commonwealth Fund, n.d.).

In contrast to fee-for-service healthcare delivery in the United States, the English healthcare system is publicly financed. In 2014, the UK allocated 9.9% or 10% of its GDP to healthcare. The NHS accounted for 79.5% of this expenditure. Taxation is the main source of UK public healthcare financing whereas limited amounts come from national insurance (payroll deductions, similar to the United States). Patients who use the NHS as a private insurer are obliged to make copays that add to NHS revenue. In general, the UK has universal healthcare. Every private resident in England has access to care and is automatically enrolled in the NHS system. Most care is free. The same services are provided to nonresidents with European Health Insurance. Like the U.S. system, undocumented non-European immigrants have access limited to emergency and infectious-disease services.

In contrast to the United States, private health insurance does not contribute significantly to the healthcare system. In 2015, about 10.5% of the UK population had private health insurance. In comparison to U.S. public health coverage, the NHS is funded through tax revenue that is a combination of employer-sponsored programs supplemented by 11% private voluntary insurance, suggesting that 3.94 million policies were in effect at the beginning of 2015. Unlike the difficulty of navigating the private insurance system in the United States, UK private health insurance provides convenient access to care. The downside, however, is that the majority of policies have no plan for mental health, maternity services, emergency services, and general practice, in contrast to the ACA, which mandates private insurance companies carry these services.

The quality of patient care in the market-based fee for service is not favorable compared to countries that have universal health systems. Fee-for-service does not protect patients from financial hardship. Instead, it exposes many low-income individuals to financial catastrophic, which could be a direct result of medical costs. In 2017, the United States had $10,209 per capita GDP healthcare expenditure, which was more expensive than $4,246 in the UK, $4,902 in France, $5,385 in The Netherlands, and $4,826 in Canada (OECD, 2018). U.S. per capita expenditure on healthcare does not positively correlate with a healthy lifespan.

The years of potential life lost in 2015 in the United States was 4,721 per 100,000 people in contrast to 2,997 in the UK, 2,266 in Japan, and 3,022 in Canada (OECD, 2018). Although potential life lost is an indicator of health-system performance, it should be applied cautiously, considering the population size of each country. In 2016, the United States had an average life expectancy of 78.6 years, differing from 84.1 in Japan, 81.2 in the UK, 81.1 in Germany, 82.4 in Sweden, and 81.9 in Canada. The infant mortality was recorded at 5.9 per 1,000 live births in the United States, 4.7 in Canada, 2.7 in Japan, and 3.4 in Germany, as of 2016 (OECD, 2018). Although these indicators need to be cautiously interpreted and applied based on country-specific demographics, they do indicate that the EHS model of health-system quality patient care might not be effective as in countries that have a compulsory health system.

In the U.S. healthcare system, CMS is a government agency responsible for government insurance: Medicare, Medicaid, and CHIP. Medicare in the U.S. health system is a federally run program that provides health insurance for individuals aged 65 and older, and people with a disability that are deemed eligible for coverage. In collaboration with each individual state, CMS administers Medicaid and CHIP, serving the limited-income population (The Commonwealth Fund, n.d.). Medicaid insurance provides access to individuals who are not covered through employer-based sponsorship and fall in the limited-income category. Medicaid provision is in the state purview in that individual states decide whether to expand Medicaid. In the U.S. health system, Medicare is financed through payroll tax deductions, similar to social health insurance in Germany, premiums, and federal tax revenue; in contrast, Medicaid is financed through federal and state tax revenue.

The operational framework of WHO endorsing a sustainable health system comprises a team-based approach from the private sector, government agencies, nongovernmental organizations, and voluntarism. Access to healthcare can be a fundamental right in some countries and more transactional in others (Ogden, 2012, pp. 49–50). In population health systems, the end goal is to reduce the impact of morbidity, mortality, and disability through community approaches. In contrast, the personal health system aims to improve the livelihood of individuals through healthcare delivery at a personal level. Its goal is to reduce mortality, morbidity, and disability through individual patients (Ogden, 2012, p. 50). The personal health system provides these efforts on the personal or individual level rather than through a general approach. Health systems can take the form of any of the following: entrepreneur, welfare-oriented, comprehensive, and socialist (Ogden, 2012, p. 50). In the United States, healthcare delivery is decentralized compared to the centralized system in the UK.

In the U.S. EHS, market reactions can influence delivery and insurance coverage. This system is predominately owned by private entities that control the production of facilities, equipment, and personnel. The choice of coverage affects this system. In this system, individual healthcare coverage can be employer-based and not mandatory. Healthcare coverage in this model could be purchased through the market by individuals with an out-of-pocket payment scheme (Ogden, 2012, p. 52; The Commonwealth Fund, n.d.). In contrast, the welfare-oriented model is more universal than choice because it guarantees all residents access to care (Ogden, 2012, p. 52). Everyone in this system must have healthcare insurance. The welfare-insurance system is mostly funded by employers and contributions from nonprofit insurance plans, also called sickfunds (Ogden, 2012). Private ownership dominates this system. However, it is self-regulated with government oversight and aligns with the tenets of egalitarianism, sharing, and redistribution of wealth through taxation.

If the healthcare market fails to protect patients from financial hardship, government intervention could result from malfunctions in allocation, stabilization, and distribution of resources. If the market fails to allocate goods and services for effective and efficient use, the government intervenes. Market failure can come from sellers and buyers, production, and consumption fatigue. Market failure could results from sellers' monopolies or monopsonies (Ogden, 2012, p. 54). Public goods are meant for public use to benefit the group or individuals. This sense of public consumption, framed as nonrivalry, does not exclude anyone, regardless of their status. Rather, companies compete in sales of private goods. The level of consumption is determined by payment (Ogden, 2012, p. 54).

In most cases, publicly funded healthcare systems get their sources from tax revenue. The government has the ability to increase income taxes, corporate taxes, value-added taxes, and in rare cases, payroll taxes that are not for healthcare (Ogden, 2012, p. 54) to sponsor healthcare programs that are crucial to population health. The tax-funded model of healthcare can be seen in countries like Canada, Italy, Spain, the Scandinavian countries, and the U.S. Medicaid program (Ogden, 2012, p. 55).

In a similar way, SHI is financed by payroll tax deductions and supplemented by tax revenue. Named after its founder, Germany Chancellor von Bismarck, in this system employers and employees share the cost. It is limited to formal employment, which is challenging for countries with low GDP, particularly those in Southeast Asia and Sub-Saharan Africa with a large pool of informal employment sectors (Ogden, 2012, p. 55). The SHI system is implemented in Germany, France, Israel, Belgium, The Netherlands, Japan, and Switzerland, and minimally in Latin and Central America. SHI is delivered by a mandatory mechanism through quasiprivate insurers or social insurers rather than the government. The Medicare portion of the U.S. healthcare system is a model of SHI funded through a combination of payroll taxes, individual cost-sharing, and general revenues (Ogden, 2012, p. 55).

In the United States, the Great Depression brought an increase in private insurance. Employer-sponsored insurance is similar to SHI, but also differs in many ways. It is voluntary, tax-deductible, and not transferable. Employer-sponsored insurance began during the Great Depression as a way for hospitals to earn income through prepaid insurance rather than taxable compensation for workers. Financing healthcare sources also include donations from charitable organizations internally that could provide bilateral or multilateral aid. Financing health systems from low GDP countries are largely from grants, loans, donations of goods and services, WHO, and World Bank multilateral aid programs. Bilateral aid passes from rich to poor. Global health financing was estimated to range from $15 billion in 2000 to $45 billion in 2006 (Ogden, 2012, p. 56).

Rationale

The quality of patient care in the global health system is an important component of health-service delivery. The quality of patient care and patient-centered care should be tailored so providers engage in the patient's world to recognize and diagnose illness through patient experience (McWhinney, 1989, as cited in Mead and Bower, 2000). The quality of patient-centered care should be approached from the patient's perspective such that the provider–patient encounter becomes conversational, with the patient taking the lead in expressing personal experiences (Byrne & Long, 1976, as cited in Mead & Bower, 2000). The quality of patient care should include 1) exploring the disease and the illness experience; 2) understanding the whole person; 3) finding common ground regarding management; 4) incorporating prevention and health promotion; 5) enhancing the doctor–patient relationship; and 6) "being realistic" about personal limitations and issues such as the availability of time and resources (Stewart, Brown, and Weston et al., 1995a, as cited in Mead & Bower, 2000). Despite the emergence of patient quality care as crucial to health-services delivery, universal access to care does not conform even across countries.

In the United States, the majority of insurance market-based institutions are privately operated with minimal public, federal, and local-government entities. The U.S. health system lacks a single-payer system and individual states have the discretion to regulate insurance companies. The inability of the state to regulate the complicated insurance system can engender financial catastrophic for patients. A major component of the health system should be to improve the health status of its population. The health system should aim to protect citizens from financial hardship due to medical costs (Fried & Gaydos, 2002, p. 36). A sustainable health system should not create financial crisis or hardship for those who seek care.

An optimal healthcare financing system should substantiate a revenue-generating system that provides care for people without exposing them to risk factors such as poverty (Fried & Gaydos, 2002). Individuals should have access to care through public or private services. According to the WHO (2007) Framework, healthcare financing should have 1) adequate funds for effective use for healthcare financing, 2) out-of-pocket spending should alternate with prepaid-insurance schemes like insurance risk pooling, 3) the poor should have access to finances and not experience financial hardship that is a direct result of health costs, 4) the system should be evaluated to maintain efficient use of resources, 5) the financial system should be transparent through information sharing, and 6) information should be readily available on health-system financing (Fried & Gaydos, 2002, p. 36).

Similar to fee-for-service market-based insurance schemes in the United States, regulated private insurance in The Netherlands is provided through nonprofit healthcare organizations that are competitive, but allow individuals to choose their insurance company (Seervai et al., 2017). The employer–employee pooling system is redistributed to insurers according to risk factors to minimize the risk of picking only healthy enrollees. A private provider provides services to the population according to their need and is reimbursed by insurance companies, similar to the U.S. Medicare reimbursement system. In contrast to U.S. choice insurance, Netherlands insurance is compulsory for all residents, except when exempted. In most cases, those who are underprivileged or in the low-income category have access to care subsidized by government funds to compensate for premium payment. It is at the government's discretion to determine the insurance package. In this system of care, consumers pay a deductible or out-of-pocket amount. In contrast, services that includes primary care, maternity care, home nursing care, and care for children are deductible-free. Similar to the UK system, the Dutch system allows people to add private insurance at personal cost.

Although every country has a health system—welfare, NHS, mixed system, or EHS, exploratory data analysis confirms that health systems are not unique. The NHS, such as in the UK, is compulsory for all residents and is an ideal choice for a health system that seeks to improve the quality of patient care. Although social health insurance in Germany, France, Japan, and other countries with universal access to care is convenient for high-GDP economies, it might not be suitable for low-GDP economies because it could undermine the quality of patient care in these countries.

Healthcare systems around the world differ significantly. Although universal coverage predominates in high-GDP countries, the United States remains the only country without universal care. The landmark ACA legislation, passed in 2010, was a major step forward for the United States to ensure its population has equitable access to healthcare. Despite being law, the ACA continues to face many legal challenges. Although 32 million Americans received insurance from the ACA marketplace, it has faced several challenges to contain costs and protect people with financial hardship who seek care. Unlike universal coverage in the global market, the effectiveness of the market-based fee-for-service health system in the United States remains

National Healthcare Expenditures

The NHE is big in U.S. healthcare. According to the CMS (2018), the annual NHE is now estimated at 18% of the U.S. GDP. CMS has been reporting on key indicators affecting the U.S. health spending since 1960s, including healthcare goods and services, public-health initiatives, government administration, net cost of health insurance, and investments pertinent to healthcare (CMS, 2018). CMS has also reported data on funding sources and enterprises directly sponsoring these sources. It has estimated that annual healthcare spending increased by 4.3% in 2016, bringing it to an unseemly $3.6 trillion or $10,348 per capita in 2018.

Figure 21: Annual percent change in GDP and national healthcare expenditures (1987–2016)

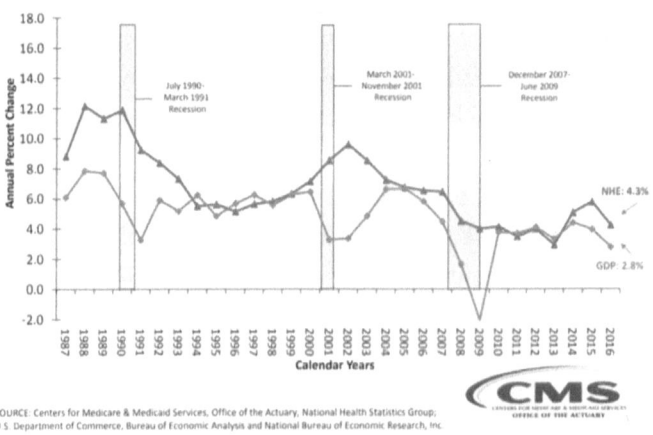

SOURCE: Centers for Medicare & Medicaid Services, Office of the Actuary, National Health Statistics Group; U.S. Department of Commerce, Bureau of Economic Analysis and National Bureau of Economic Research, Inc.

While hospital costs rose in 2015, the growth was slower in 2016 at about 5.7% (CMS, 2018). Similarly, physician- and clinical-services cost sharing growth was lower in 2016 than in 2015. Despite these subtle differences, physician and clinical cost was nearly $664.9 billion of the NHE budget. In addition to physician and medical cost sharing, prescription-drug cost sharing in the NHE budget was $328.6 billion in 2016. This growth was about 1.3% lower than the large jump of 8.9% seen in 2015. Among the sources for the NHE, the central government bears a significant burden. Providing nearly 28.3% of NHE through sponsor programs followed by households (28.1%). In contrast, private insurance covers roughly 19.9% healthcare costs, followed by state and local governments (16.9%), and private revenue (6.7%).

The United States has long had a fragmented and fragile healthcare system. Since the inception of Medicare and Medicare in the 1960s, providing an equitable healthcare delivery system has been heavily subsidized. In the 21st century, where chronic diseases have taken a substantial toll on the population, subsidies are not an optimal way to solve this broken system. A recent report suggests that nearly 50 million American adults are struggling with chronic pain (CDC, 2018). Chronic medical conditions will continue to affect the U.S. population as it ages. A robust system must be in place to meet the many challenges expected in the near future.

Although the ACA brought the U.S. healthcare system under a single umbrella, the cost of care is expected to continue rising (CMS, 2018). By 2026, NHE will be $5.7 trillion. The growth of healthcare spending will outpace GDP growth by 1.0%, so NHE could reach 28% of GDP by 2026. Demographic and economic transitions will influence this trend as enrollment shifts from private insurance to Medicare due to an aging population and as the cost of medical goods and services continues to rise (CMS, 2018). This shift will be absorbed by Medicare and Medicaid, growing by 7.4% and 5.8% per year, respectively. While the ACA has been under constant threat from the current administration, it would be a costly mistake to do away with the individual mandate, which would affect insurance enrollment. It is notable that economic growth might impact the insurance market some, offsetting this growth. Nearly 91.1% of the U.S. population was insured in 2016, whereas the CMS projected 89.3% by 2026 due to GDP growth.

PHE has increased over time in the United States. This is due to a system that includes a widening the wealth gap between the top 1% and the bottom 50%. Taxpayers are at risk, particularly the so-called working families who suffer the consequences and associated costs of disease. The top 1% or even 20% enjoy optimal health, but the bottom 20% or 50% suffer. What is missing from the United States' so-called wealth is that when the rich are sick, they only worry about the disease and not the monetary cost because they can afford it. They are worried about the course of the disease and, in most cases, they receive the best care. In contrast, when the poor are sick, they focus on the course of the disease and the cost. Most Americans are brainwashed into believing the loud message coming from their political leaders. The U.S. healthcare system is a fantasy of Island. Only those who can find their way will be rescued. Perhaps the United States could learn from Canada, the United Kingdom, Germany, France, or Turkey. These countries have not only an affordable healthcare system, but also patient-centered care.

As the U.S. population ages, PHE will continue to rise. For example, in 2012, the PHE for seniors aged 65 and above was nearly $18,988. Understanding this figure is crucial. The new generation should be aware that this figure could even grow higher. The PHE for individuals age 65 and over was $6,632 more than for working-age adults and nearly five times more than the average cost spent on a child (CMS, 2018). In 2012, the average PHE for females was $8,315, 22% higher than for males ($6,788).

NHE does vary by state. While the NHE grew on average by 3.9% from 2009 through 2014, North Dakota experienced a far more significant increase than any other state, 6.9%. In contrast, Rhode Island's spending grew very little, averaging nearly 2.5% (CMS, 2018). The highest PHE in the nation was seen in California, collectively about $295 billion. In 2014, California's PHE made of up 11.5% of the national total PHE. This might not be a surprise considering that California is the most populous state in the nation. Gigantic PHE was also seen in New York, Texas, Florida, and Pennsylvania. Due to its conventional history of managing healthcare, Wyoming's PHE was about 0.2% of U.S. PHE in 2014. These states' historically low portion of U.S. healthcare expenditure could be due to their small populations. Figure 22 presents the NHE as a share of GDP from 1987 to 2016.

Figure 22: National health expenditures as a share of GDP, 1987–2016

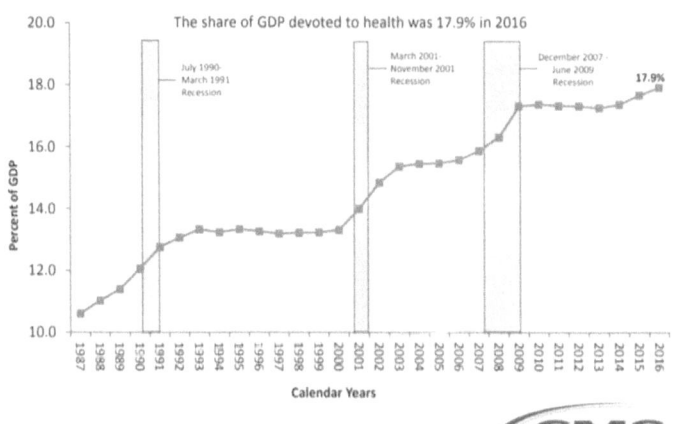

SOURCE: Centers for Medicare & Medicaid Services, Office of the Actuary, National Health Statistics Group; U.S. Department of Commerce, Bureau of Economic Analysis and National Bureau of Economic Research, Inc.

As shown in Figures 21 and 22, NHE continued to rise as a share of GDP from 1987 to 2009, just before the adoption of the ACA in 2010. While the ACA provided coverage to nearly 32 million uninsured Americans, it did not prevent NHE from rising. From 2010 to 2016, NHE grew to 17.9% of GDP, suggesting the need for additional measures if healthcare spending is to be contained. Figure 23 suggests that private insurance significantly influences the U.S. healthcare system. In 2016, an estimated 196.4 million Americans had private or employer-sponsored insurance, whereas Medicaid and Medicare combined had just 127 million enrollees. Since the implementation of the ACA, the number of uninsured has dropped from over 44 million of just over 28 million people. Despite 28 million people being uninsured, indicating that the ACA is far from perfect, Americans at least have the freedom to choose healthcare. People are no longer rejected for having preexisting conditions. Despite the individual mandate's repeal by the Republican Congress in 2018, nearly 92% of the U.S. population had insurance in 2018.

CONTEMPORARY ISSUES IN THE U.S. HEALTHCARE DEBATE

Figure 23: Enrollment in private health insurance, Medicaid, and Medicare, and the uninsured (levels in millions)

	2013	2014	2015	2016
Private Health Insurance	187.6	192.8	196.3	196.4
Employer Sponsored	169.2	169.8	172.2	173.1
Individual	20.0	24.5	25.6	24.8
Marketplace		5.4	9.0	10.0
Medicaid	58.9	65.9	69.1	71.2
Medicaid Newly Eligible		6.6	9.6	11.4
Medicare	51.3	52.8	54.3	55.8
Uninsured	44.2	35.5	29.5	28.6
Insured Share of Population	86.0%	88.8%	90.8%	91.1%

NOTE: Enrollment estimates are not mutually exclusive. The estimate of Marketplace enrollment reflects average monthly enrollment and not enrollment at the end of the year.

SOURCE: Centers for Medicare & Medicaid Services, Office of the Actuary, National Health Statistics Group.

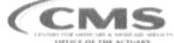

Although healthcare choice is a significant milestone in the U.S. healthcare debate, containing cost could be hard without compulsory universal healthcare. Per capita healthcare expenditures have continued to rise even though the ACA has played a significant role in reducing that growth rate. Factors that account for growth are age and sex of the population, medical prices, and residual use and intensity. Figure 24 indicates that in 2016 per capita healthcare grew 3.5%.

Figure 24: Health spending per capita growth rates, 2004–2016

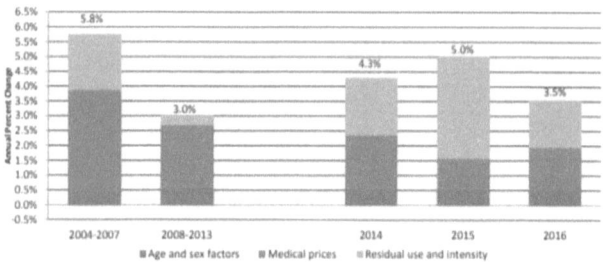

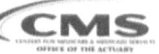

NOTES: Medical price growth, which includes economywide and excess medical-specific price growth (or changes in medical-specific prices in excess of economywide inflation), is calculated using the chain-weighted national health expenditures (NHE) deflator for NHE. "Residual use and intensity" is calculated by removing the effects of population, age and sex factors, and price growth from the nominal expenditure level.

SOURCE: Centers for Medicare & Medicaid Services, Office of the Actuary, National Health Statistics Group.

While the NHE $3.6 trillion budget might continue to rise, it is vital to understand where the bulk of the money goes. According to data in Figure 25, an estimated 32% of the nation health dollar went to hospital care in 2016. Physician and clinical spending made up 20% while another 20% went to other spending. Other spending here seems rather vague for such a large category, considering the United States has such a wasteful healthcare system.

Figure 25: Cost sharing of health dollar, 2016

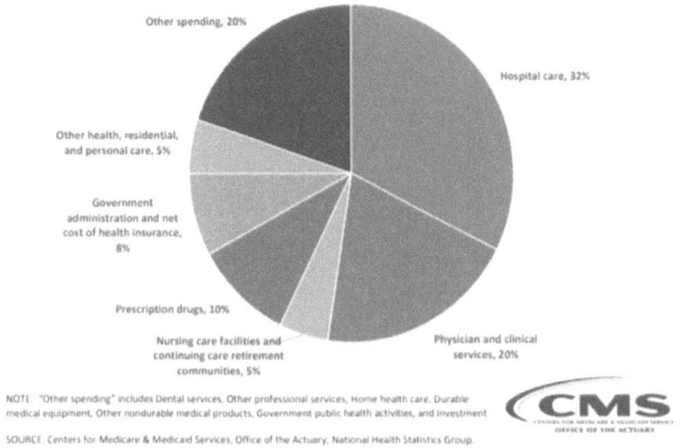

- Hospital care, 32%
- Physician and clinical services, 20%
- Other spending, 20%
- Prescription drugs, 10%
- Government administration and net cost of health insurance, 8%
- Other health, residential, and personal care, 5%
- Nursing care facilities and continuing care retirement communities, 5%

NOTE: "Other spending" includes Dental services, Other professional services, Home health care, Durable medical equipment, Other nondurable medical products, Government public health activities, and investment

SOURCE: Centers for Medicare & Medicaid Services, Office of the Actuary, National Health Statistics Group.

Prescribing drugs took the lead in annual growth spending on healthcare in 2015 and 2016. In 2015, prescription drugs grew about 8.9% (Figure 26). Debate on healthcare reform should take into account the manipulating influence from the mega insurance and pharmaceutical companies that are driving the cost of healthcare. Annual spending for hospital care in 2016 was $1.1 trillion. Hospital spending increased by 4.7% in 2016, which was slower than the 6.0% rise in 2012 (Figure 27).

Figure 26: Annual growth in spending by type of goods and services, 2015–2016

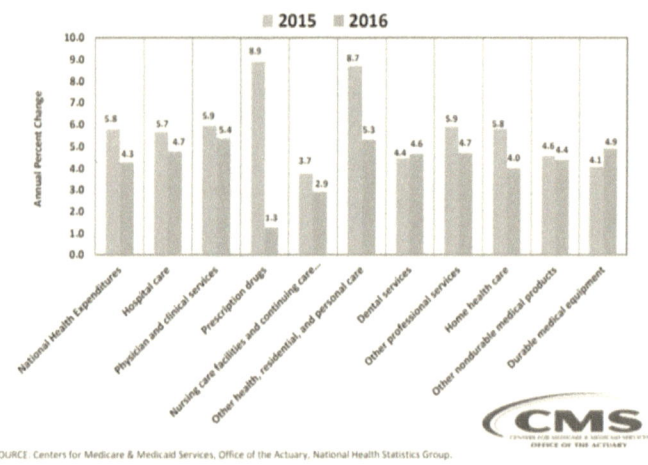

Figure 27: Annual growth in hospital spending, 2012–2016

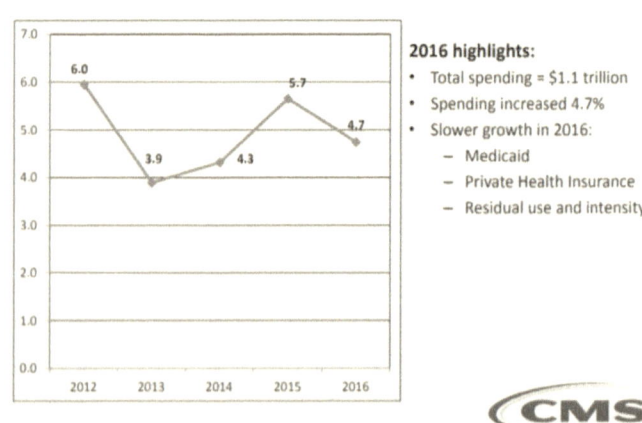

2016 highlights:
- Total spending = $1.1 trillion
- Spending increased 4.7%
- Slower growth in 2016:
    - Medicaid
    - Private Health Insurance
    - Residual use and intensity

As highlighted in Figure 28, the annual physician spending in 2016 was $664.9 billion. As shown in Figure 25, physician and clinical services represented about 20% of the NHE annual budget in 2016. The spending includes Medicare, Medicaid, and residual use and intensity. Although physician and clinical spending growth slowed by 0.5% from 2015 to 2016, it is expected to grow as the NHE budget continues to rise.

Figure 28: Annual growth in spending by physician and clinical services, 2012–2016

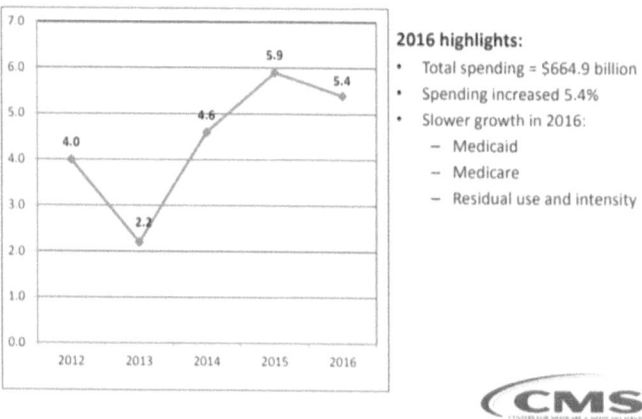

SOURCE: Centers for Medicare & Medicaid Services, Office of the Actuary, National Health Statistics Group.

Figure 29: Annual growth in retail prescription spending, 2012–2016

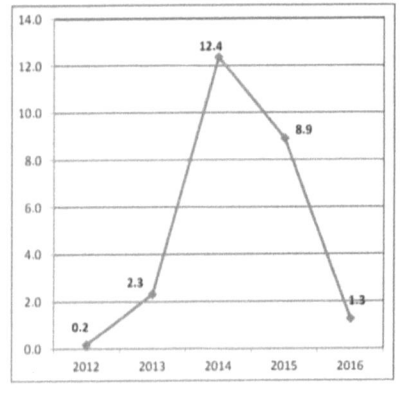

2016 highlights:
- Total spending = $328.6 billion
- Spending increased 1.3%
- Slower growth in 2016:
  - Fewer new drugs approved
  - Slower growth in brand name drugs
    - Decline in spending for hepatitis C drugs

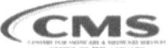

SOURCE: Centers for Medicare & Medicaid Services, Office of the Actuary, National Health Statistics Group.

Figure 30: Sources of national health expenditures, 2016

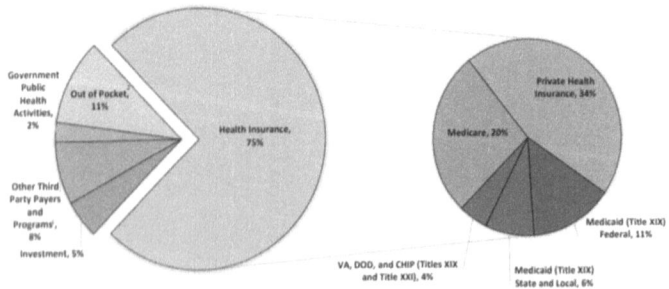

[1] Includes worksite health care, other private revenues, Indian Health Service, workers' compensation, general assistance, maternal and child health, vocational rehabilitation, Substance Abuse and Mental Health Services Administration, school health, and other federal and state local programs.
[2] Includes co-payments, deductibles, and any amounts not covered by health insurance.
Note: Sum of pieces may not equal 100% due to rounding.

SOURCE: Centers for Medicare & Medicaid Services, Office of the Actuary, National Health Statistics Group

Figure 31: Private health insurance: Growth and enrollment, total and per-enrollee expenditures, 2012–2016

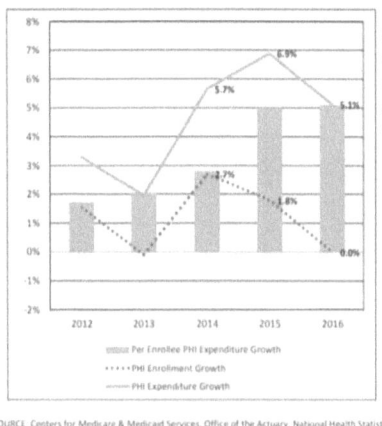

2016 highlights:
- Total Spending = $1.1 trillion
- Spending increased 5.1%
- Enrollment growth slowed
- Per enrollee increased 5.1%
  - Slower growth in retail prescription drug spending
  - Slower growth in hospital spending
  - Faster growth in net cost

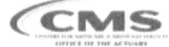

SOURCE: Centers for Medicare & Medicaid Services, Office of the Actuary, National Health Statistics Group

Figure 32: Medicare: Growth and enrollment, total and per-enrollee expenditures, 2012–2016

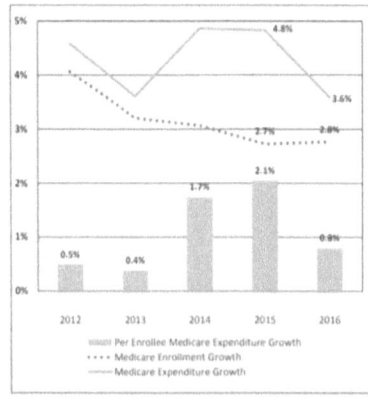

2016 highlights:
- Total Spending = $672.1 billion
- Spending increased 3.6%
- Enrollment growth fairly stable
- Per enrollee increased 0.8%
  - Slower growth in Prescription drug spending
  - Slower growth in Physician and clinical services spending
  - Slower growth in Nursing home spending

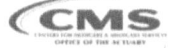

SOURCE: Centers for Medicare & Medicaid Services, Office of the Actuary, National Health Statistics Group

Figure 33: Medicaid: Growth total, federal, state, and local expenditures, 2012–2016

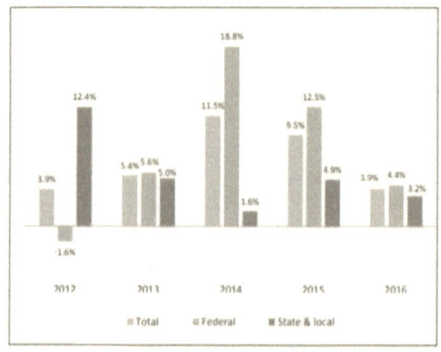

SOURCE: Centers for Medicare & Medicaid Services, Office of the Actuary, National Health Statistics Group.

Figure 34: National health expenditures: Distribution and growth by type of sponsor

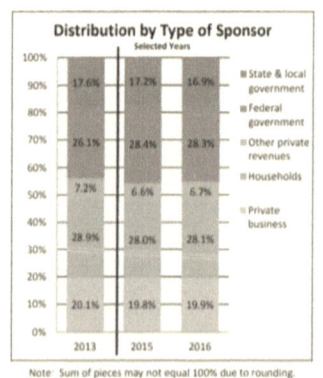
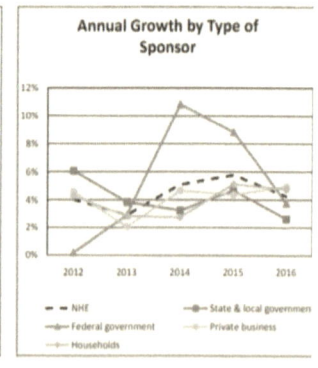

SOURCE: Centers for Medicare & Medicaid Services, Office of the Actuary, National Health Statistics Group.

Figure 35: Where the national health expenditures are spent

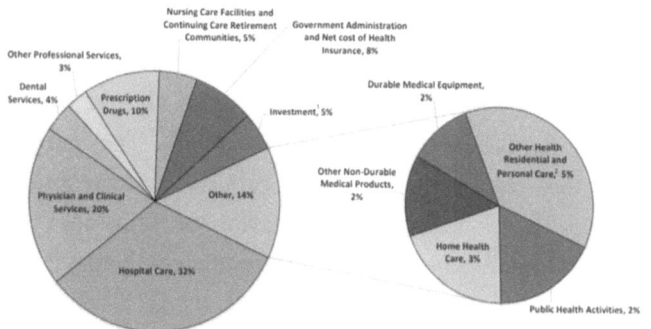

[1] Includes Noncommercial Research and Structures and Equipment.
[2] Includes expenditures for residential care facilities, ambulance providers, medical care delivered in non-traditional settings (such as community centers, senior citizens centers, schools, and military field stations), and expenditures for Home and Community Waiver programs under Medicaid.
Note: Sum of pieces may not equal 100% due to rounding.

SOURCE: Centers for Medicare & Medicaid Services, Office of the Actuary, National Health Statistics Group.

The Way Forward

Reform in the U.S. healthcare system must be rejuvenated at the micro and macro levels. At the micro level, healthcare facilities (hospitals, clinic, and managed care) must reform their leadership capacity to employ leaders in top positions who are well informed about an institutional transformation that includes Medicare, Medicaid, commercial, and private insurance. These transformations are vital to patient care and are deeply embedded in the U.S. Healthcare debate. Mastery of leadership at the micro level is vital to pushing the healthcare system forward to success or backward to failure. Studies have demonstrated transformational leadership to be more productive with respect to teamwork, commitment, staff satisfaction, and followers' self-efficacy (Alloubani et al., 2014; Delmatoff & Lazarus, 2014).

Alloubani and colleagues (2014) argued that strong leadership contributes significantly to organizational success. While an organized leadership might conform to the organization's principles, adapting to change can be challenging (Delmatoff & Lazarus, 2014). The research shows that leadership requires a process of development and growth, sanctioning the adoption of emotional and behavioral intelligence to cope with several challenges facing the healthcare industry (Delmatoff & Lazarus, 2014; Green et al., 2013; Longenecker & Longenecker, 2014).

At the macro level, Congress should clearly and coherently adopt a bipartisan policy that does not aim at dismantling the Affordable Care Act; rather, Congress should make necessary changes as has been done with Medicare. Several factors must be considered to achieve optimal reform: drug and other medical costs, partisanship, medical-education costs, and government efficiency.

First, drugs are extremely expensive in the United States due to pharmaceutical company greed. U.S. healthcare costs are skyrocketing due to a poorly regulated and fragile market that allows thousands of for-profit insurance companies and providers affect patient care. Pharmaceutical companies set high costs for drugs, and insurance companies decide how much patients can pay for copay, coinsurance, premiums, and deductibles.

Often patients are in limbo with huge unpaid medical bills. U.S. doctors are highly paid but spend less than 45 minutes per visit to examine each patient. Doctors should use EHR to swiftly document patient contact and save valuable time (Seymour, Frantsvog, & Graeber, 2012). In some instances, unnecessary laboratory tests are ordered due to patient-rights and legality concerns that have evolved in the healthcare system. Imaging—such as computed tomography (CT) scans, magnetic resonance imaging (MRI), and X-Rays—are extremely expensive and not every patient can afford it. Some patients who need these services are among the supposed working class. They make too little to afford insurance, but too much to qualify for most subsidies.

Second, the AMA and AHA must make a rational decision. From the 1930s to the present, these two powerful associations have been instrumental in bringing the U.S. healthcare system to where it is today. Physicians in the United States fear that a government-mandated universal healthcare system would jeopardize their income. In the 1940s, the AMA and AHA rose up to oppose President Harry S. Truman attempt to solve the healthcare crisis. In contrast to Franklin D. Roosevelt's 1935 enactment of SS, as World War II was winding down in 1945, Truman's administration shifted its attention to the national crisis of health insurance for all Americans (American College of Healthcare Executives, n.d.). Truman's proposal on healthcare for all Americans drew heavily criticism from the AMA and the AHA: The bill was too socialized and liberalized since the bill could give patients the ultimate freedom to choose their own providers. Most critics argued that a universal healthcare policy seems too socialist while others have completely dismissed the idea, claiming that it cannot work in the United States. Although not perfect, the ACA passed into law during President Obama's administration brought the U.S. healthcare system closer to universal access.

In a remarkable reversal, the AMA and AHA supported a bill proposed by Senators Lister Hill (D-AL) and Harold Burton (R-OH), the 1946 Hill-Burton Act, that introduced unprecedented subsidies for hospitals and nursing facilities and became an integral part of the U.S. healthcare system. Instead of national health insurance for all Americans, efforts were redirected to care for senior citizens. The platform approach for subsidy supported by the AMA and AHA remained unchanged while millions of American were trapped without healthcare until the adoption of the ACA in 2010. While subsidies offered hope for some patients, they were heavily directed to Medicare patients. The U.S. population has seen the chilling effects of chronic disease. Subsidies might not be workable in the long run as long as the AMA and AHA resist any rational bill consistent with medical ethics in support of a universal healthcare for all.

Third, medical schools must be reasonable with tuition and fees. In an unusual move in 2018, New York University announced it would offer free tuition for its medical students for the 2018–2019 academic school year (NYU Langone Health, n.d.). Whether this is sustainable should be explored. The high cost of medical school has been a barrier for college students wishing to pursue a medical career. As the U.S. population continues to grow, it will require more health professionals, particularly in primary care. If the cost of medical school continues to grow at its current rate, the United States risks losing it high rank in the biomedical fields. It will have to depend on foreign scientists, who receive higher education at low cost in their native countries.

Fourth, the federal government must be smart. The United States has many resources, but it has been very wasteful. The government should invest more in education, reduce student loan burdens, and make medical schools attractive to college students. The need to train biomedical scientist has never been stronger. Physicians will be skeptical about their salary and oppose any affordable care for all if they have accumulated student loans that would take them 20–30 years to pay. That is insane.

Finally, if the system fails to address these problems, concerned citizens should take to the street and demand their government to provide them with affordable care. While the ACA should be maintained, it is a healthcare system. There are thousands of insurances in the ACA market, each one of these insurance companies charges different premiums, deductibles, and coinsurance. Premiums and deductibles are too high. Most so-called working-class families still cannot afford these costs. Although the ACA has brought the U.S. insurance system under a single umbrella, many nuances must be fixed to reduce costs. No one will fix this but a government of the people, by the people, and for the people. If the U.S. government fails its aging population faced with the risk of chronic disease, it runs the risk of a healthcare crisis. The healthcare system will not collapse, but the price will go out of control and society will be more unequal than ever.

REFERENCES

Alloubani, A.M et al. 2014. Effects of Leadership Styles on the Quality of Services in Health Care. European Scientific Journal, 10(18), 118–129.

American College of Healthcare Executives. (n.d.). History of Health Insurance in the United States. Available at: http://www.ache.org/pubs/morrisey2253_chapter_1.pdf. Accessed September 2, 2018.

CDC. 2018. Health and Economic Costs of Chronic Diseases. Available at: https://www.cdc.gov/chronicdisease/about/costs/index.htm. Accessed September 29, 2018.

Centers for Medicare & Medicaid Services. 2018. National Health Expenditure Data Fact Sheet 2016. Retrieved July 25, 2018, from https://www.cms.gov/research-statistics-data-and-systems/statistics-trends-and-reports/nationalhealthexpenddata/nhe-fact-sheet.html

—2018. Centers for Medicare & Medicaid Services. National Health Expenditure Data Fact Sheet 2016. Retrieved July 25, 2018, from https://www.cms.gov/research-statistics-data-and-systems/statistics-trends-and-reports/nationalhealthexpenddata/nhe-fact-sheet.html.

—Center for Disease Control and Prevention (CDC). n.d. Sortable Risk Factors and Health Indicators: US Population Estimates in 2014. Available at: https://sortablestats.cdc.gov/#/demographics. Accessed October 9, 2018.

CIA World Factbook. 2018. North America: United States. Retrieved July 30, 2018, from https://data.worldbank.org/country/united-states.

—Deaths and Mortality: Number of deaths for leading cause of deaths. 2017. Available at: https://www.cdc.gov/nchs/fastats/deaths.htm. Accessed October 9, 2018.

—Sortable Risk Factors and Health Indicators. 2015. Available at: https://sortablestats.cdc.gov/#/detail. Accessed October 9, 2018.

—Sortable Risk Factors and Health Indicators. N.d. The 33 indicators are categorized in 4 groups. Available at: https://sortablestats.cdc.gov/#/summary. Accessed October 9, 2018.

Delmatoff, J., & Lazarus, I. 2014. The Most Effective Leadership Style for the New Landscape of Healthcare. Journal of Healthcare Management, 59(4), 245–249.

Dieleman, J.L; Baral, R; Birger, M et al. (2016). US Spending on Personal Health Care and Public Health, 1996-2013. Jama-Journal of The American Medical Association, 316(24), 2627-2646.

Green, A.E et al,. 2013. Transformational Leadership Moderates the Relationship Between Emotional Exhaustion and Turnover Intention Among Community Mental Health Providers. Community Mental Health Journal, 49(4), 373–379.

Chen, J.G; Zou. B.; Shuster, J. (2017). Relationship Between Patient Satisfaction And Physician Characteristics. Journal of Patient Experience, 4(4), 177-184.

CIA the World Factbook. 2018. North America: United States. Retrieved July 30, 2018, from https://data.worldbank.org/country/united-states. Downing, N. L; Bates, D.W; Longhurst, C.A. 2018. Physician Burnout in the Electronic Health Record Era. Are We Ignoring the Real Cause? Annals of Internal Medicine, 169 (1); 50-51

Donaldson, C. & Bryan, S. 2012. Compulsion: The Key to US Health Care Reform. Journal of Health Services Research & Policy, 17(2); 106-109.

Downing, N. L; Bates, D.W; Longhurst, C.A. 2018. Physician Burnout in the Electronic Health Record Era. Are We Ignoring the Real Cause? Annals of Internal Medicine, 169 (1); 50-51

Echouffo-Tcheugui, J.B; Bishu, K.G; Fonarow, G.C; Egede, L.E. 2017. Trends in healthcare expenditure among US adults with heart failure: The Medical Expenditure Panel Survey 2002-2011. 186, 63-72.

Fried, B. J. & Gaydos, L. M. (2012). World health systems: Challenges & perspectives. Chicago: Health Administration Press. ISBN: 978-156793420-5.

Gulliford, M et al. (2002). What does 'access to health care' mean? Journal of Health Services Research & Policy, 7(3), 186-188.

International Monetary Fund. 2018. World Economic Outlook (WEO) Database. Retrieved July 25, 2018, from http://comstat.comesa.int/IMFWEO2018Apr/imf-world-economic-outlook-weo-database-april-2018.

Kaiser Family Foundation. 2016. Health Insurance Coverage of the Total Population. Available at: https://www.kff.org/other/state-indicator/total-population/?currentTimeframe=0&sortModel=%7B%22colId%22:%22Location%22,%22sort%22:%22asc%22%7D. Accessed October 9, 2018.

—Health Insurance Coverage of the Nonelderly (0-64) with Incomes below 100% Federal Poverty Level (FPL). 2016. Available at: https://www.kff.org/other/state-indicator/nonelderly-up-to-139-fpl/?currentTimeframe=0&sortModel=%7B%22colId%22:%22Location%22,%22sort%22:%22asc%22%7D. Accessed October 9, 2018.

—Distribution of the Nonelderly Uninsured by Age. 2016. Available at: https://www.kff.org/uninsured/state-indicator/distribution-by-age-2/?currentTimeframe=0&sortModel=%7B%22colId%22:%22Location%22,%22sort%22:%22asc%22%7D.

Accessed October 9, 2018.

—Distribution of the Nonelderly Uninsured by Family Work Status. 2016. Available at: https://www.kff.org/uninsured/state-indicator/distribution-by-employment-status-2/?currentTimeframe=0&sortModel=%7B%22colId%22:%22Location%22,%22sort%22:%22asc%22%7D.

Accessed October 9, 2018.

—Distribution of the Nonelderly Uninsured by Race/Ethnicity. 2016. Available at: https://www.kff.org/uninsured/state-indicator/distribution-by-raceethnicity-2/?currentTimeframe=0&sortModel=%7B%22colId%22:%22Location%22,%22sort%22:%22asc%22%7D. Accessed October 9, 2018.

Kindig, D. A. & Isham, G. (2014). Population health improvement: A community health business model that engages partners in all sectors. Frontiers of Health Services Management, 30(4), 3-20.

Kayes, K.M & Galea, S. 2016. Setting the agenda for a new discipline: Population health science. American Journal of Public Health, 106(4), 633-634.

Lee, M.H; Schuur, J.D; Zink. B.J. (2013). Owning the Cost of Emergency Medicine: Beyond 2%. Annals of Medicine, 62(5), 498-505.

Longenecker, C.O., & Longenecker, P.D. 2014. Why Hospital Improvement Efforts Fail: A View from the Front Line. Journal of Healthcare Management, 59(2) 147–157.

Maeda, H. 2018. The Rise of the Current Mortality Pattern of the United States, 1980-1930. American Journal of Epidemiology, 187(1), 639-646.

Martin, D et al. 2018. Canada's Universal health-care system: achieving its potential. The Lancet, 391(10131), 1718-1735.

Mead, N; Bower, B. (2000). Patient-Centeredness: a conceptual framework and review of the empirical literature. Social Science & Medicine 51, 1087-1110.

Mebsesan S. L. 2015. Population Health. An Analysis of the Definition and a Measurement of the Concept. Bulletin of the Transilvania University of Brasov. Series VII: Social Sciences, 8(2), 135-144.

Morrison, I. 2014. The Second curve of Population Health. Trustee, 67(5), 17.20.

New York Medical School: https://med.nyu.edu/education/md-degree/md-affordability-financial-aid/cost-attendance access September 9, 2018

Organization for Economic Cooperation and Development. 2018. Gross Domestic Product (GDP). Retrieved July 23, 2018, from https://data.oecd.org/gdp/gross-domestic-product-gdp.htm#indicator-chart.

—Organization for Economic Corporation and Development (OECD). 2018. Selected Indicators for United States. Available at: https://data.oecd.org/united-states.htm. Accessed October 10, 2018.

—Organization for Economic Cooperation and Development. 2016. Income Inequality. Available at: https://data.oecd.org/inequality/income-inequality.htm. Accessible September 15, 2018.

—Organization for Economic Cooperation and Development. 2015. Poverty Rate. Available at: https://data.oecd.org/inequality/poverty-rate.htm#indicator-chart. Accessible November 15, 2018.

—Health Spending. 2018. Available at: https://data.oecd.org/healthres/health-spending.htm. Accessed October 10, 2018.

—Doctors. 2018. Available at: https://data.oecd.org/healthres/doctors.htm#indicator-chart. Accessed October 10, 2018.

—Nurses. 2018. Available at: https://data.oecd.org/healthres/nurses.htm#indicator-chart. Accessed October 10, 2018.

Institute for Healthcare Improvement (IHI). n.d. A Primer on Defining the Triple Aim. Available at: http://www.ihi.org/resources/Pages/Publications/PrimerDefiningTripleAim.aspx. Accessed October 10, 2018.

Petrou, P; Samoutis, G; Lionis, C. 2018. Single-payer or a multipayer health system: a systematic literature review. Public Health, 163, 141-152.

Polikowski, M; Santos-Eggimann. (2002). How Comprehensive are the basic packages of health services? An international comparison of six health insurance systems. Journal of Health Services Research & Policy, 7(3), 133-142.

Seervai, A; Shah, A; & Osborn, R. 2017. "How Other Countries Achieve Universal Coverage," To the Point, The Commonwealth Fund.

The Commonwealth Fund. N.d. The U.S Healthcare System. Available: https://international.commonwealthfund.org/countries/united_states/. Accessed October 14, 2018.

The World Bank. 2018. United States. Retrieved July 30, 2018, from https://data.worldbank.org/country/united-states.

United Nations Human Rights. 2017. Statement on Visit to the USA, by Professor Philip Alston, United Nations Special Rapporteur on extreme poverty and human rights*. Available at: https://www.ohchr.org/EN/NewsEvents/Pages/DisplayNews.aspx?NewsID=22533. Accessed November 15, 2018.

Wallace, J. (2014). 3-pillar approach to integrated population health management. Healthcare Financial Management, 68(4), 68-72.

World Health Organization. N.d United States of America Statistics. Retrieved July 30, 2018, from http://www.who.int/countries/usa/en/.

www.ingramcontent.com/pod-product-compliance
Lightning Source LLC
Chambersburg PA
CBHW020440220526
45464CB00002B/783